Speech and Deafness

Speech and Deafness

A Text for Learning and Teaching

By
Donald R. Calvert
Director, Central Institute for the Deaf
Associate Professor of Audiology, Washington University

and
S. Richard Silverman
Director Emeritus, Central Institute for the Deaf
Professor of Audiology, Washington University

Alexander Graham Bell Association for the Deaf
Washington, D.C.

HV
2471
.C3

Copyright © 1975 by
The Alexander Graham Bell Association for the Deaf, Inc.
First Edition

The Alexander Graham Bell Association for the Deaf, Inc.
3417 Volta Place, N.W., Washington, D.C. 20007, U.S.A.

Library of Congress Catalogue Card Number 75-226-02
ISBN 0-88200-070-5

To
Rae Calvert and Sally Silverman,
longstanding members of the
company of learners and teachers.

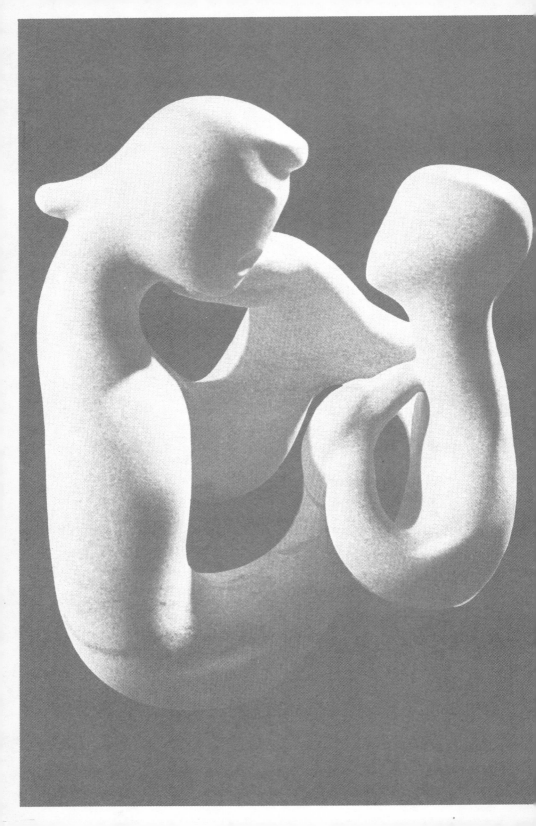

The awesome task for those of us engaged daily in teaching speech is to recapitulate for our deaf children the evolution of humankind's extraordinary and unique achievement—spoken language. Contemplate, if you will, the vast symbolic structures built by the human race and transmitted by sounds; what a feat, as Lewis Mumford points out in his "Myth of the Machine," of abstracting, associating, memorizing, recognizing, recalling, that at first must have demanded "strenuous collective effort!" No technological triumph surpasses its grandeur and its power.

S. Richard Silverman
The Volta Review, March 1974.

Preface

An indispensable requirement for effective teaching is the recognition that the responses of students govern the development of instructional practices. Our book constitutes an attempt to satisfy that requirement. It grows out of many years of experience in listening and reacting to students, colleagues, and deaf persons, and, in turn, develops our ideas and our suggestions for them about learning and teaching speech. In a very real and significant sense, all of us who have positive convictions about the value of communication by speech are members of a company of enthusiastic learners. In this spirit our book delineates a point of departure for continued learning rather than arrival at a final destination. It is a beginning, not an end. We predict with confidence that as we continue to learn, revision and elaboration will be inevitable. We would be disappointed if it turned out to be otherwise.

To all from whom we have learned we express our gratitude. Their "responses" stimulated the preparation of the pages that follow. We are singularly indebted to Daniel Ling of the School of Human Communication Disorders, McGill University, Montreal, Canada, for the chapter on Amplification for Speech, and to Jean S. Moog and Ann V. Geers of the staff of Central Institute for the Deaf for permission to append the current version of their "Scales of Early Communication Skills for Hearing Impaired Children." We thank, too, Audrey A. Simmons-Martin, James D. Miller, and Randall Monsen, all of the Institute staff, for contributing specific items as noted in the text.

We trust that those who benefit from the use of the material in this book will have the same rich satisfaction that its authors have had not only in presenting the material but, perhaps more importantly, in contributing toward enabling a deaf child to acquire the precious skill of spoken language. This will be reward enough for our efforts.

Donald R. Calvert
S. Richard Silverman

St. Louis, Missouri
October 1975

viii

Table of Contents

List of Tables		x
List of Figures		xi
Introduction		1
Chapter I	Speech and Its Production	6
Chapter II	Learning and Teaching Speech	40
Chapter III	Amplification for Speech	64
Chapter IV	Instructional Analysis of Consonants and Vowels	89
Chapter V	Developing Speech	147
Chapter VI	Beyond Development of Speech	173
Appendix	Scales of Early Communication Skills for Hearing Impaired Children	197
Bibliography and Suggested Readings		202
Index of Names		237
Index of Subjects		241

List of Tables

Table 1.   Phonetic consonant symbols of Northampton, IPA, and dictionary markings, with key words.   10

Table 2.   Phonetic vowel symbols of Northampton, IPA, and dictionary markings, with key words.   11

Table 3.   The proportion of times each of 20 Northampton symbols represents the designated vowel sounds in 7,500 common words.   14

Table 4.   Estimated ratings of sensory feedback information for consonants.   25

Table 5.   Estimated ratings of sensory feedback information for vowels.   26

Table 6.   Correlation of motor and language development.   43

Table 7.   Percent of hearing impaired students with specified additional handicapping conditions by age group, United States: 1971-72 school year.   44

Table 8.   Estimated ratings of sensory instructional possibilities for consonants.   59

Table 9.   Estimated ratings of sensory instructional possibilities for vowels.   59

Table 10.   Digest of sensory aids applied to the primary factors of speech (auditory, visual, tactile, and kinesthetic senses).   60-61

Table 11.   Rank ordering of groups of phonemes by ease of development, made by teachers of deaf children.   161

Table 12.   Guide to term of initial approach and age at assessment.   169

Table 13.   Rank ordering of phonemes by frequency of correction needed.   178

Table 14.   Percentage of deaf and normal speech samples meeting the criterion of 70% agreement at several levels of articulatory complexity.   191

List of Figures

Figure 1. Recurring situations in which speech can be functional. 3

Figure 2. Northampton consonant chart. 12

Figure 3. Northampton vowel chart. 13

Figure 4. Diagram of structures used in speech production. 16

Figure 5. Stages of children's dentition. 17

Figure 6. Top view diagram of the tongue in its normal relaxed position and in positions of a narrow point and a broad front. 19

Figure 7. Vowel diagram showing relative tongue position for vowels. 21

Figure 8. Consonant sounds ordered by their manner and place of production. 23

Figure 9. Relative position of contact of the tongue for implosion of breath for **k** preceding vowels **ee** and **oo**. 27

Figure 10. Phrasing as shown by intensity variation. 37

Figure 11. A gross composite estimate of the information features of speech related to severity of hearing loss. 38

Figure 12. Areas of concern in learning and teaching speech. 41

Figure 13. The relation between distance and sound pressure level of speech in a non-reverberant room with an ambient noise level of 50 dB. 68

Figure 14. Spectrogram of a sentence. 70

Figure 15. Spectrogram of **s** and **sh**. 73

Figure 16. Effect of amplified speech. 79

Figure 17. Response of typical body-worn hearing aid. 80

Figure 18. Some steps of language development. 155

All photos by Ken Nicolai were provided courtesy of the Central Institute for the Deaf, St. Louis, Missouri.

Introduction

Throughout the recorded history of the education of the deaf the desirability of equipping the deaf person with spoken language has seldom if ever been questioned. From the 16th and 17th centuries—which marked the period when literature about the education of the deaf began to emerge—through the period of the development of influential movements, to the present day, issues, values, and methods about teaching speech have commanded the interest and attention of writers, teachers, deaf persons, and observers of the field (185). Of course, the continuing controversy about modes of communication that are emphasized in the education of the deaf persists, and, here and there, this causes variation in the significance that is placed on instruction in speech for the deaf. Nevertheless, none of the proponents of one or another view advocates elimination of teaching speech. We hope that what we have included in this book can be incorporated beneficially in whatever mode of communication is prominent in instruction and associated activities.

As we have said, teachers vary considerably in the emphasis they place on the teaching of speech, ranging all the way from teachers for whom the teaching of spoken language is a central focus to those whose attitudes toward teaching speech are crystallized in such comments as, "It's nice to do it, if you can get it, but don't spend too much time on it." This range of attitudes usually results in varying outcomes ranging from the production of intelligible speech to what amounts to just a string of unintelligible grunts or snorts. This last result discourages those who would spend more time on teaching speech. Attitudes which evolve into a spectrum of firmly held convictions seem to grow out of what in the modern managerial idiom we would call the *cost benefits* of teaching speech. These convictions have fed on themselves and—in many contexts where benefits in relation to expended efforts

1

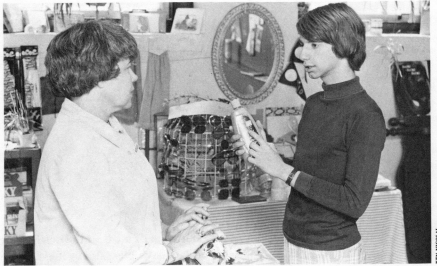

Shopping—speech is functional.

have been judged, for whatever reason, to be insufficient—have unfortunately contributed to the denigration of the teaching of speech. In such situations there is very little reinforcement of attempts in classrooms, clinics, and homes—let alone in the general environment—to encourage or to improve speech by deaf persons.

Obviously the fact that we have undertaken to write this book underlines our conviction that the development of spoken language for deaf children and its improvement for deaf adults is worth every effort we can put forth. We are aware that even the best efforts may not ensure complete intelligibility of all deaf persons' speech in all situations, but as suggested in Figure 1, there are recurring communicating situations in which speech can be importantly functional. In a sense, the recurrence provides "auditory training" to the listener. The continuing aim should be the extension of the areas of understanding listeners. To reduce or abandon our best efforts in teaching speech to deaf persons is to deny them the opportunity for an achievement unique to man—the development of an acoustic code that enables a human being to communicate with his fellow human being in a distinctive way that is not possible through any other mode of communication.

Our aim in this book is to improve the competency of those who would take the teaching of speech to deaf children seriously, with the hope that their results may be improved. This, in turn, should reinforce their own efforts and consequently their own enthusiasm for the activity. In the pages that follow we have attempted to concentrate on the task of teaching and learning speech through the eyes of the person in whom the professional responsibility resides, namely the teacher, and, to some extent, supportive persons and parents. We have used the term "teacher" to apply to instructional personnel in schools and to speech pathologists and audiologists who are involved in programs for hearing impaired persons.

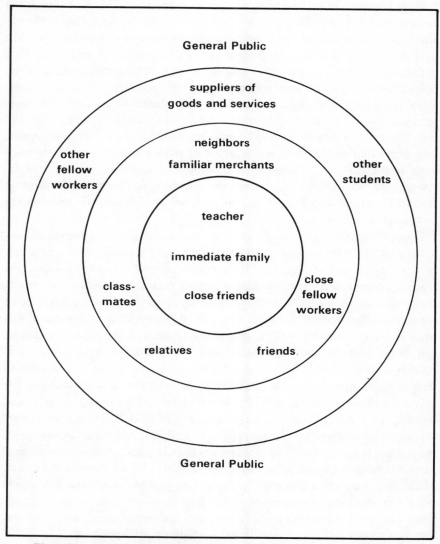

Figure 1. *Recurring situations in which speech can be functional.*

What we have presented is based primarily but not exclusively on our own experience as teachers and as teachers of teachers. It is our chief credential for tackling the problem in the first place. This is essentially an "applied" book, though not a "manual." Its optimum use will be facilitated by continuing experience and direct application with students. We are not only aware, we are *convinced*, that a teacher's competence will be enhanced by her knowledge of the contributions to her task from related bodies of knowledge. We believe, however, that these subjects are adequately treated elsewhere in the professional and scientific literature. We have drawn on them only to the extent that they are directly and demonstrably relevant to developing speech in deaf individuals. Because indifference to the obvious, but essential, can be a pedagogical pitfall, we have here and there restated and condensed material from these sources as handy references or brief refreshers, some shamefully elementary, for the teacher. The inclusion of fundamental anatomy and physiology and some conventional orthographic symbol systems are examples of this. The point is that we wish to avoid being diverted from our main purpose into exposition and even critical analysis of related areas, particularly since we hope the sources contained in our bibliography accomplish this effectively. Among the bibliographic items are some which we have selected for annotation to illustrate the kinds of helpful material available in the professional and scientific literature.

It would be presumptuous of us to state that we have treated our subject exhaustively. We have covered as much as we believe is pertinent, or necessary, to serve as a point of departure for a practitioner. We hope to enhance the teacher's *power to analyze the task of speech instruction and to plan procedures that follow logically from the analysis.* After all, children differ, environments differ, and teaching and instructional styles differ. The value of this book to the teacher will be commensurate with what she brings to the task by way of her own attitudes, knowledge, and skill. These stress an attitude that reflects a strong conviction about the worthwhileness of teaching speech to deaf persons; knowledge that underlines and strengthens the possibility for improvement in a teacher's ability, which should be a lifelong process; and building on a rational set of procedures applied to skilled instruction. Furthermore, all of this must be expressed in the context of the school in which the teacher practices her skills. This means that, in a school, we do *not* depend just on a designated specialist, helpful as such may be, to improve the speech of children, but rather that *every teacher is also a teacher of speech.* We cannot stress this point too strongly. We believe that attention to speech is not just a matter of something that is given for x number of minutes per day, but that it pervades all of the instructional procedures and activities.

We have searched diligently and extensively for an organizing scheme for this book that would by itself contribute to the achievement of its aim. After a good deal of cutting, pasting, modifying, eliminating, and adding, what follows represents our best current judgment. There is more than an expected amount of repetition and redundancy, as, for example, in the emphasis in different contexts on the use of residual hearing. This is deliberate in order to drive home our points, and it is also helpful for the teacher who may wish to pass over certain parts and plunge immediately into others.

Our text follows what we believe is an orderly, logical sequence. We start with speech and its production, refreshing our reader on anatomy, physiology, and some of the related acoustics. Then we consider learning and teaching speech, emphasizing general principles that lead to specific kinds of recommendations and suggestions. We then move on to Dr. Ling's chapter on acoustic amplification in teaching speech.We have included this as a separate chapter because of the number of children in schools and classes for the deaf who have hearing levels that command recognition in the teaching of speech. Furthermore, it makes available Dr. Ling's abundant experience in research in the use of residual hearing, its relation to acoustic phonetics, and its practical application. Recent data from the Gallaudet College Center for Demographic Studies indicate that 45% of hearing impaired children are reported to have hearing levels of 84 dB* or better in three speech frequencies. Incidentally, if the frequency of 250 Hz had been included in the calculation and a cut-off established at 90 dB, the numbers of children with hearing significant for speech development would be much greater.

Dr. Ling's chapter on amplification is followed by a detailed analysis for instruction of the phonemes and combinations of phonemes. Originally we had intended to include this in the Appendix, but it seemed to fit better here. We progress to the task of developing speech, and here we suggest "strategies" to the teaching of speech that encompass traditionally discrete but overlapping methods. Chapter VI underlines the fundamental point that speech must not only be developed, but must be improved, corrected, and maintained. We hope that the bibliography will stimulate and add to the intellectual and professional sense of accomplishment the teacher derives from her work.

Throughout we have used the terms *deaf* and *hearing impaired* interchangeably. Agreement on the precise definition of these terms is still not universal. For convenience of style we have referred to the student as *he* and the teacher as *she*. We trust that activists in the "role of the sexes" movement will not treat our decision too harshly.

---

*Except where otherwise specified, all references to dB may be understood to be ISO calibration.

CHAPTER I

Speech and Its Production

Speech may be studied from many points of view. It may be analyzed from a physical base, relating the body's vibrating and resonating systems to the frequency, intensity, and duration of the sounds of speech. Considered physiologically, the emphasis may be on interaction of muscles, cartilage, and bone, or on neurological activity such as excitation, transmission, integration, and response of the body's nervous system. Viewed psychologically, speech is concerned with personality, self-expression, and such processes as motivation, attention, perception, recognition, and memory. Speech also has an obvious socio-linguistic base as the prime vehicle for symbolically expressing meaning through language and as an important medium through which humans interact among themselves. How speech develops in individuals and how it has come to be one of mankind's distinctive achievements continues to command the attention and energy of investigators and practitioners.

For our purposes, as stated in the Introduction, we select material from those complex and richly stocked areas which are pertinent to our task. It is necessary that we organize our exposition around the analysis of those aspects of speech production that experience suggests are most useful in teaching children to talk. Various "models" for teaching and learning speech are now being investigated. Their validation and usefulness may result in changes in conceptualization of our task. For the present, however, we believe it is

6

timely and pragmatic to organize our material in this chapter dealing with speech production around the primary factors influencing intelligibility. These are **articulation, voice,** and **rhythm**.

ARTICULATION

The process of shaping the breath stream from the larynx out through the mouth to form the speech sounds of language is called articulation. In talking, speech sounds do not follow one another as separate and distinct units like beads on a string. Nor do they flow forth in infinite variety, inseparable and unrecognizable. Each language has a finite number of speech sounds which recur within a limited range of variations.

Phonemes

The essential elements of these recurring sounds, recognized by listeners as the code signals which give meaning to speech, are called **phonemes**. Phonemes are abstractions, somewhat like an averaging, of those sounds which actually occur in connected speech. In the words *tea, cat, stay*, and *cattle*, we recognize a recurring common sound represented by the letter "t." We call this the phoneme **t**.* Yet in each of these words, the **t** is produced somewhat differently. In *tea*, the **t** is produced with the tongue tip on the gum ridge behind the front teeth and is exploded with audible breath just before beginning the vowel sound. The **t** in *cat* is typically a stop made without explosion or with very slight explosion of breath. In *stay*, the **t** stops the flow of breath but is not exploded as it is in *tea*. In *cattle*, the tongue remains on the gum ridge and the audible release is made laterally around the sides of the tongue. These and other variations of producing the phoneme **t** are called its **allophones**. These are phonetic variations in the place of articulation of the speech sounds within an utterance.

There are other common variations in the production of phonemes which may occur without changing meaning. The rhythm of speech may change the force with which a sound is produced to make its duration longer or shorter. In various regions of the world and among some cultural and ethnic groups where English is spoken, people speak with variations of the language called **dialects**. Dialects include variation in the production of some speech sounds, such as the southern United States "drawl" which lengthens and proliferates vowel sounds, or, as in the northeastern United States, the apparent omission of the **r** following a vowel as in *park*. Further variations are added in com-

---

*Throughout this book Northampton symbols, printed in boldface, will be used to represent phonemes. See Figures 2 and 3 for charts of these symbols.

paring the speech of those in cities and of those in rural areas of the same region. Of course, each speaker produces variations in speech sounds in his unique way, adjusting for the size and shape of his own speech mechanism.

Relation to meaning is an essential feature of the phoneme. When boundaries are exceeded in varying the production of a phoneme, it may be recognized as another phoneme (and thus change the meaning of a word) or not be recognized at all. For example, when the **t** sound is made with very little audible explosion where explosion is expected, listeners may recognize it as the phoneme **d** (try producing the word *tie* with no audible explosion of the **t**). When the **-i-** in *bit* is produced with the mouth open wide, the listener is likely to hear other vowel sounds such as the **-e-** in *bet* or the **-a-** in *bat*.

Orthographic Systems

To communicate about the phonemes of our language, we need a standard system of written symbols. In some languages, such as Spanish, the letters of standard spelling almost always have the same sound associated with them. But English is not so fortunate. It does not have a simple symbol-sound correspondence. Perhaps, this is because the English language developed from a mixture of the languages of Europe. Anglo-Saxon, derived primarily from Germanic dialects, was mixed with French and influenced by the Scandinavian languages of northern Europe, the Romance languages of southern Europe, and classic Greek and Latin. While this agglomeration of origins enhances our facility in expressing ourselves, its spelling and pronunciation follow no consistent set of rules.

Pronunciation which is not consistently predictable from spelling leads to problems. As we encounter a new word in print we determine its approximate meaning through the context of the words and phrases around it. We also formulate a probable pronunciation, using the rules of pronunciation and spelling we have learned inductively through our constant use of the language. But quite often we are aware that a new word can be pronounced several different ways because the rules of pronunciation we have learned are not absolute.

A major problem in English pronunciation is that the alphabet does not contain enough symbols to represent the phonemes of the language. English has an alphabet of only 26 letters to represent 43 sounds. The five letters which are called vowels (*a, e, i, o, u*) must represent 18 different vowels and diphthongs. The 21 consonant letters represent 25 different consonants. There is, for example, no special letter which represents the first phoneme in *church*. A number of other phonemes are represented in spelling by a combination of two letters as in *sh, th, wh* and *ng*.

A second related problem in English pronunciation is that the letters are not always pronounced the same way. While most consonant letters represent a single sound, none of the vowel letters exclusively represents a single sound. Note how pronunciation of the letter "o" changes in these words: *ton, top, told, tomb, woman, women*. However, some systematic pronunciation is evident. The 18 vowel sounds are more frequently represented by a single vowel letter, or by a particular combination of vowel letters, than by some other letter or combination of letters. Still a third problem in English pronunciation is that a single phoneme may be represented by a number of different letter combinations. The sound of **f**, for example, may be spelled "f " (*fir*), "ff " (*differ*), "ph" (*phone*), "gh" (*rough*) or "lf " (*half*).

We now consider some of the systems that address themselves to these problems.

The International Phonetic Alphabet: To avoid the spelling irregularities within a language, the differences in spelling from language to language, and the use of written characters other than Roman alphabet symbols in some languages, the International Phonetic Alphabet (IPA) was developed. The IPA includes a number of sounds which are not typically used in English, such as the bilabial fricative sound common in Spanish (*Havana*) and the fricative **r** sound common to Middle Eastern languages. It also provides for refined transcription with supplementary symbols describing particular variations in phoneme categories. The comprehensive and analytic features of this system make it especially useful for scholarly and professional communication about language and speech. (See Tables 1 and 2.)

Visible speech symbols: Alexander Melville Bell and his son Alexander Graham Bell suggested a system of "visible speech" in 1894. In this system consonants are represented by four fundamental curves that relate to the "articulators," that is, to the back of the tongue, the top of the tongue, the point of the tongue, and the lips. The insertion of a short "voice" line in the bow of the curve changes a voiceless consonant to a voiced consonant. There is also a system for modifying a set of fundamental symbols to represent the vowels. This system is described in Bell's *The Mechanism of Speech* (8).*

Visual-tactile system: Dr. A. Zaliouk, late Director of the Institute for the Deaf in Haifa, Israel, devised a "visual-tactile system of phonetic symbolization" for teaching speech to the deaf. This system uses two categories of symbols: static and dynamic. The static symbols represent the hard palate,

*The numerals in parentheses here and throughout the text refer to numbered readings in the annotated bibliography beginning on page 202.

the tongue, the teeth, and the lips, all of which participate in various "articulatory positions." The dynamic symbols indicate movement (92).

Diacritical markings: Dictionaries use a system of diacritical markings (symbols attached to letters) to indicate pronunciation. Roman alphabet letters are used with special symbols attached to some of them to indicate their pronunciation. Common diacritical markings and dictionary symbols are shown in Tables 1 and 2.

Primary Northampton Symbol	IPA Symbol	Dictionary Diacritical Markings	Key Words
h-	/h/	h	*had, ahead*
wh	/ ʍ /	hw	*when, everywhere*
p	/p/	p	*pie, sip, stopped*
t	/t/	t	*tie, sit, sitting*
k	/k/	k	*key, back, become*
f₁	/f/	f	*fan, leaf, coffee*
th	/θ/	t͟h	*thin, tooth, nothing*
s₁	/s/	s	*see, makes, upset*
sh	/ ʃ /	s͟h	*she, fish, sunshine*
ch	/t ʃ/	c͟h	*chair, such, teacher*
w-	/w/	w	*we, awake*
b	/b/	b	*boy, cab, rabbit*
d	/d/	d	*day, mud, ladder*
g	/g/	g	*go, log, begged*
v₂	/v/	v	*vine, give, every*
th	/ð/	t̶h̶	*the, smooth, bother*
z	/z/	z	*zoo, size, lazy*
zh	/ʒ/	z͟h	*measure, vision*
j	/dʒ/	j	*jam, edge, enjoy*
m	/m/	m	*meat, team, camera*
n	/n/	n	*new, tin, any*
ng	/ŋ/	n͡g	*song, singer*
l	/l/	l	*low, bowl, color*
r	/r/	r	*red, bar, oral*
y-	/j/	y	*yes, canyon*
x			*box, taxi*
qu			*queen, liquid*

Table 1. *Phonetic consonant symbols of Northampton, IPA, and dictionary markings, with key words.*

Northampton symbols: At the Clarke School for the Deaf in Northampton, Massachusetts, dissatisfaction with the Bell symbols as a teaching device led Alice Worcester, a teacher, to develop symbols taken from the Roman alphabet, which she published in 1885. They were revised and organized into systematic charts in 1925 by Caroline Yale. These symbols have been very popular with teachers of the hearing impaired because they help students with word pronunciation. Throughout this book we shall use the primary symbols for phonetic transcription of phonemes.

The principle of the Northampton symbol system is to use as primary symbols either the alphabet letters most frequently used for particular sounds in speech (as **p, f, s̀, n**) or symbols which are not most common but almost invariably represent particular sounds when they occur in writing (as **k, ee, a-e** as in *name,* **aw** as in *law*).

Secondary symbols reflect the irregular relation between written letters and sounds. For example, "k" is the primary symbol for the **k** phoneme (as in **k**ind). The letter "k" almost invariably represents the **k** phoneme, but it is not as commonly used to represent the sound **k** as is the letter "c" (as in *can*).

Primary Northampton Symbol	IPA Symbol	Dictionary Diacritical Markings	Key Words
oo¹	/u/	o͞o	*boot, too*
oo²	/ʊ/	o͝o	*book, could*
aw	/ɔ/	ô	*awful, caught, law*
ee	/i/	ē	*east, beet, be*
-i-	/ɪ/	i	*if, bit*
-e-	/ɛ/	e	*end, bet*
-a-	/æ/	a	*at, mat*
a(r)	/ɑ/	â(r)	*odd, father, park*
-u-	/ʌ/	u	*up, cup*
-u-	/ə/	ə	*above, cobra*
ur	/ɝ/	er	*urn, burn, fur (General U.S.)*
a-e	/eɪ/	ā	*able, made, may*
i-e	/aɪ/	ī	*ice, mice, my*
o-e	/oʊ/	ō	*old, boat, no*
oi	/ɔɪ/	oi	*oil, coin, boy*
u-e	/ju/	yo͞o	*use, cute, few*

Table 2. *Phonetic vowel symbols of Northampton, IPA, and dictionary markings, with key words.*

However, the letter "c" may have the sound of $\overset{1}{s}$ (as in *city*) or of **sh** (as in *ocean*), as well as the sound of **k**. The letter "c" is therefore a secondary symbol for the **k** sound, but it also is used as a secondary spelling for the $\overset{1}{s}$ sound. Learning the primary and secondary spellings of the Northampton symbol system can be a great help in learning to pronounce words, even though this system does not account for all irregularities of our spoken language.

Figures 2 and 3 contain charts of the Northampton symbols. In the consonant chart the left column is occupied by breath (unvoiced) consonants, the second column by the voiced forms of the same sounds, and the third column by the nasal sounds. Horizontally the consonants are arranged according to the place of articulation. A dash following a letter indicates that the sound is initial in a word or syllable.

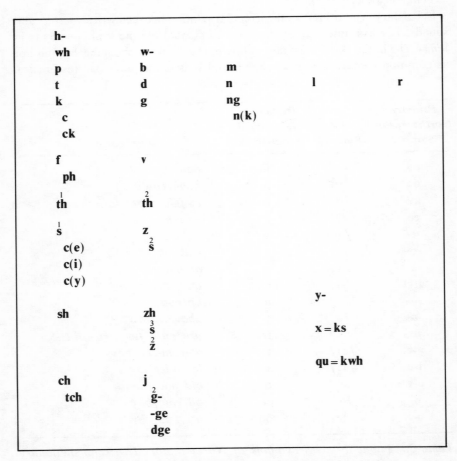

Figure 2. Northampton consonant chart.

In the vowel chart the upper line contains the back round vowels (those modified chiefly by the back of the tongue and the rounded aperture formed by the lips). The second line contains the front vowels (those modified chiefly by arching the front of the tongue). The lowest line contains the diphthongs. At the very bottom are vowelized consonants which perform the function of a vowel, constituting a syllable at the end of words.

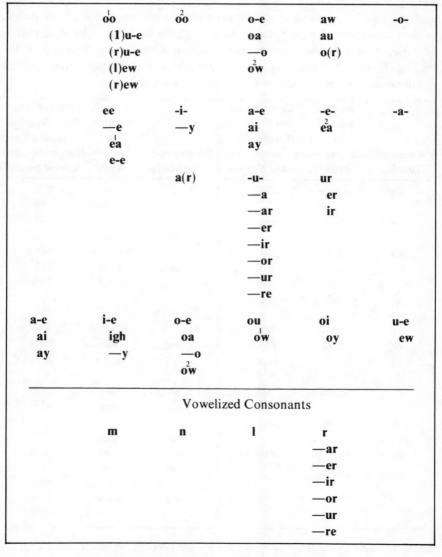

Figure 3. Northampton vowel chart.

Table 3 shows the correspondence between the spellings of some Northampton symbols and vowel sounds, based on a study of pronunciation of common words. The symbols on the left side are those which consistently represent a specific vowel sound (about 90% or more of the time). The reader encountering a new word which includes one of these vowel letters or combinations of letters could be reasonably confident of the pronunciation. On the right side are spelling symbols which do not correspond very well. The spelling "ow," for example, can be pronounced like the vowel in *low* or the vowel in *cow* with almost equal frequency. The reader would be uncertain as to which would be the correct pronunciation. Other vowel spellings in the right column offer probabilities for predicting the correct pronunciation much better than by chance, although by no means perfectly.

Northampton Symbols	Vowel Sound in Sample Word	Proportion of Time Symbol Occurs To Represent that Vowel Sound	Northampton Symbols	Vowel Sound in Sample Word	Proportion of Time Symbol Occurs To Represent that Vowel Sound
a-e	make	100%	-a-	cat	83%
				table	13%
u-e	cute	100%			
			-u-	cup	73%
aw	law	100%		unite	24%
i-e	kite	99%	ea	meat	74%
				head	24%
oi	boil	99%			
			-e-	bet	70%
oa	boat	98%		be	30%
ee	beet	96%	ou	out	60%
				rough	35%
-i-	pin	91%			
	child	9%	$\overset{1}{oo}$	boot	59%
			$\overset{2}{oo}$	cook	41%
ai	bait	90%			
			-o-	top	53%
au	caught	88%		told	40%
			ow	low	52%
				cow	48%
			o-e	home	34%
				come	66%

Table 3.   *The proportion of times each of 20 Northampton symbols represents the designated vowel sounds in 7,500 common words (239).*

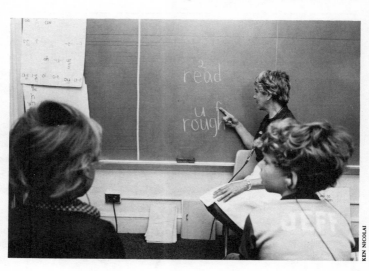

**Using
Northampton
symbols.**

None of the orthographic systems we have described satisfies all our needs for teaching speech. An ideal system of orthography would meet the following requirements: (1) The symbols would convey information about how to articulate the sounds (Bell's and Zaliouk's symbols), (2) The symbols would be free of ambiguity (International Phonetic Alphabet), (3) The system would use the written symbols of the culture (Northampton), and (4) The symbols would be perceptually feasible (all that have been cited). Obviously some of these requirements are in conflict. We believe the Northampton system offers a pragmatic accommodation for our purposes.

Place of Production

Place of production of a sound refers to that part of the speech mechanism involved directly, prominently, and specifically in the production of sound. When we refer to the "speech mechanism," we are aware that the structures that are included in it serve biological needs as their primary function. We shall allude briefly to these functions and focus on their role as providing a place of articulation. Reference to Figure 4 (page 16) will help the student in this section.

Lips (*labio-, -labial*): Their primary function is to help contain food in the oral cavity. The lips can close to stop the breath stream as in articulating **p, b,** and **m**. By approximating the lower lip and upper front teeth, the breath stream is constricted for the production of **f** and **v**. Rounding the lips and changing the degree of opening contributes to the production of **w, wh,** and the vowel sounds.

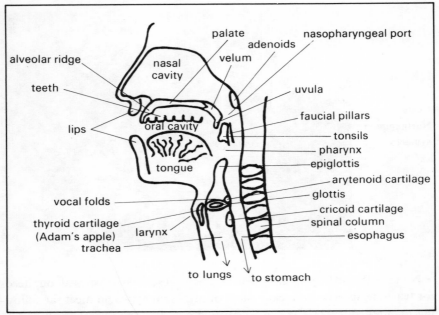

Figure 4.   *Diagram of structures used in speech production.*

Teeth (*dento-, -dental*): Their primary function is to cut and grind in chewing food. In the growing child, structures change size, shape, dominant function, and relation to other elements. A good example is the developing dentition, shown in Figure 5 (184). The deciduous teeth, sometimes called the "milk" or "baby" teeth, erupt during a period of from 6 months to 2 years of age to include 20 teeth, 10 in the upper jaw (maxilla) and 10 in the lower jaw (mandible), arranged in symmetrical sets of 5 teeth on each side. Beginning from the midline, they are: central incisor, lateral incisor, canine (or eye tooth), first molar, and second molar. Beginning at about age 6 years, the deciduous teeth are replaced with 32 permanent teeth, 16 in the upper and 16 in the lower jaw, arranged in symmetrical sets of 8 teeth on each side. Beginning from the midline, these are: central incisor, lateral incisor, canine, first bicuspid (having two sharp points, sometimes called a premolar), second bicuspid, first molar, second molar, and third molar (or "wisdom" tooth). The sides of the tongue pressed against the molars help direct the breath stream toward the front of the mouth as in **sh**. The lower lip approximates the upper front teeth to constrict the breath stream for **f** and **v**; the tongue similarly approximates the upper incisors for the **th** and **th**. The approximated upper and lower front teeth provide friction surfaces for the **s, z, sh,** and **zh**.

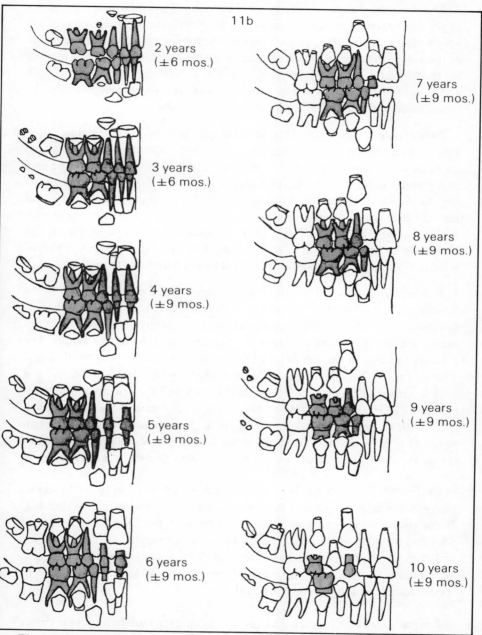

Figure 5. *Stages of children's dentition. Deciduous teeth are shown in dark tint, permanent teeth in white. From the chart, "Development of the Human Dentition," I. Schour & M. Massler. American Dental Association, 211 East Chicago Ave., Chicago, Ill. 60611.*

Alveolar ridge (*alveolo-, -alveolar*): This is the gum ridge just behind the upper front teeth. The tongue presses against the alveolar ridge to stop the breath stream for the **t, d,** and **n**. Pressing the tongue point against the center of the ridge permits the breath stream to escape on both sides of the tongue for the **l**. The tongue tip approximates the alveolar ridge in formation of the **s** and **z**; the front of the tongue at a greater distance from the ridge forms the constriction of the breath stream for the **sh** and **zh** sounds.

Palate (*palato-, -palatal*): This, sometimes called the "hard palate," is the structure separating the oral from the nasal cavity, extending from the alveolar ridge to the velum. Its primary purpose is to help contain food in the oral cavity and provide a hard superior (upper) surface for the process of swallowing. As the superior surface of the oral cavity, the palate contributes to vowel resonance. It helps to direct the breath stream toward the front of the mouth for consonant articulation. The back of the tongue presses against the back of the palate in the production of **k, g,** and **ng**. The tip of the tongue is lifted toward the palate, just behind the alveolar ridge, to help form the **r**.

Velum (*velo-, -velar*): The velum, sometimes called the "soft palate," is the structure just posterior to the palate. It raises to help close the nasopharyngeal port, thus separating the oral from the nasal cavity. The *uvula* is an appendage extending inferiorly from the posterior midline of the velum. The primary purpose of the velum is to keep food from entering the nasal cavity. The velum, by helping to close the nasopharyngeal port, helps direct the breath stream to the oral cavity for articulation and for primarily oral resonances as in vowel sounds. When the velum is relaxed and the port opened, the breath stream can enter the nasal cavity for predominantly nasal resonance as in **m, n,** and **ng**. The back of the tongue presses against the back of the palate and front portion of the velum in the production of **k, g,** and **ng**.

Oral cavity (*oro-, -oral*): This cavity extends from the lips to the throat or pharynx. Its primary purpose is to contain food for chewing and swallowing. It can also receive inhaled and exhaled air but does not have the filtering and warming capacity of the nasal spaces. It acts as a resonating cavity for voice and channels the breath stream out the mouth for sounds other than **m, n,** and **ng**. Changes in its size and shape are largely responsible for articulation of speech sounds and their perceptual features.

Tongue (*lingua-, -lingual*): The tongue is a highly mobile muscular organ arising from the floor of the oral cavity. Its primary purpose is to direct food to the back of the oral cavity in the process of swallowing. Its five landmarks, the *point*, the *tip*, the *front*, the *middle*, and the *back*, are very important to

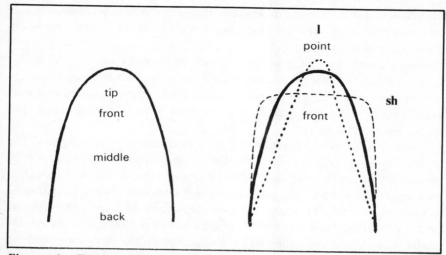

Figure 6. *Top view diagram of the tongue in its normal relaxed position (left) and in positions of a narrow point and a broad front.*

speech sound articulation. Figure 6 shows these landmarks as the very front edge of the tongue is narrowed or broadened to form the normal tip, the narrowed point, and the broadened front.

The tongue can narrow and point, as it does for the **l**, or it can present a broad front surface as it does in production of **sh**. Its tip and back sections can be elevated independently of each other. It can form a central groove to direct the breath stream as it does for **s**, or the tip can be elevated and drawn back (retroflexed) toward the middle of the oral cavity as in **r**. It can close off the oral cavity and quickly release compressed breath as it does in **t** and **k**.

Pharynx (*pharyng-, -pharyngeal*): The pharynx is posterior to the nasal cavity (the naso-pharynx), the oral cavity (the oro-pharynx), and, to a lesser extent, the laryngeal cavity (the laryngo-pharynx). The naso-pharynx and oro-pharynx are separated by the ***nasopharyngeal port*** (which can be closed by the combined actions of the velum and uvula), the faucial pillars, the posterior wall of the pharynx, and masses of the tonsils and adenoids. The primary purpose of the pharynx is to direct food to the esophagus, and air to and from the trachea. It acts as a resonating cavity for voice and channels the breath stream to the oral and nasal cavities. Closure of the nasopharyngeal port results in oral resonance and helps direct the breath stream to the oral cavity for articulation of speech sounds.

Nasal cavity (*naso-, -nasal*): Extending from the nostrils to the nasopharynx, the nasal cavity is primarily designed to receive inhaled air, filter and warm it, and direct it toward the trachea. It also channels exhaled air. The nasal cavity contributes to vocal resonance and channels the breath stream out the nose for **m, n,** and **ng.**

Speech sounds may be described by their place of production, using the structures outlined above. For example, the **t** may be described as a lingua-alveolar sound (the tongue touches the alveolar ridge), the **f** as a labio-dental sound (the lip against the teeth), and the **th** as a lingua-dental sound (the tongue against the teeth).

Vowel sounds may be described by place of elevation of the tongue in the front of the mouth (as in **ee**), the back of the mouth (as in **oo**) or the middle portion of the mouth (as in **-u-**). Vowels may be further described by whether the tongue's elevation is high (as in **ee** and **oo**), low (as in **-a-** and **a(r)**) or midway (as in **-e-** and **aw**). Using the two parameters of place and height of tongue elevation, the place of production of vowels is plotted in Figure 7. Of course, vowels are also modified by the degree of mouth opening and lip rounding.

Manner of Production

Another way of describing speech sounds is by the manner in which they are produced. The flexibility of our speech mechanism permits us to produce a surprising variety of noises. We shall consider four classes of the primary manner of speech sound production: *stops, fricatives, affricates,* and *resonants.*

Stops: These are sometimes called plosives or aspirates. The primary action in their production is an interruption of the breath stream by a closure within the oral cavity. Stop phonemes include **b, p, t, d, k,** and **g.** The stop action has two phases called the *implosion* (closure) and the *explosion* (release). Both phases are important for the teacher to know about because some allophones of stop phonemes are made without the explosion phase. For example the **t** in *stop* is imploded but not exploded, while the **t** in *top* is both imploded and exploded. The rapid stopping of a preceding vowel sound by a stop consonant changes the resonance pattern of the vowel in a way unique for the position of closure of the stop, depending on whether it is at the lips (**p** and **b**), the alveolar ridge (**t** and **d**), or the velum (**k** and **g**), so that the alteration of the vowel gives the listener important information about the stop consonant which terminates it.

Fricatives: These sounds require constriction of the breath stream with audible friction for their production. They are formed by forcing the constricted air stream over the surfaces of the lips, teeth, tongue, alveolar ridge, palate, and velum. Fricative sounds include **f, v, th, th, s, z, sh, zh, wh,** and **h.** Friction

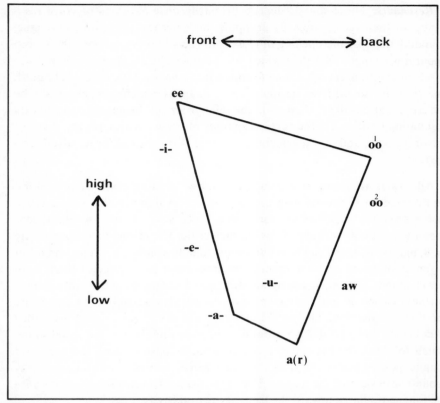

front ⟵⟶ **back**

ee

-i-   o͡o

high

↑   o͡o

-e-

↕   -u-   **aw**

↓
low   -a-

a(r)

Figure 7. *Vowel diagram showing relative tongue position, with place of tongue elevation in the mouth on the horizontal plane and degree of elevation on the vertical plane.*

may occur either with the unvoiced breath stream (as in **f, th, s, sh, wh,** and **h**), or with voicing (as in **v, th, z,** and **zh**). The term "sibilant" is sometimes applied to the **s, z, sh,** and **zh** sounds. Many other speech sounds include some degrees of friction in their production but are not dependent on friction for their perception.

Affricates: These sounds are sometimes called "stop-fricatives" because they combine a stop sound immediately followed by a fricative sound in the same syllable. During the stop portion (implosion phase) of the affricate, the fricative position is anticipated by tongue movement so that the release (explosion phase) of the stop produces the breath stream for production of the fricative portion of the affricate. Affricate sounds are **ch (t + sh), j (d + zh), x (k + s),** and **qu (k + wh).**

Resonants: These sounds depend primarily on alterations of voice resonance for their recognition. By dropping the lower jaw, elevating the tongue, rounding the lips, and opening or closing the nasopharyngeal port, the speech apparatus changes the sound which was produced at the glottis to emphasize bands of overtone energy, called **formants** (see Chapter III), which distinguish one resonant sound from another. These changes are effected physically by the combinations of (1) changes in the relative size of the pharyngeal and oral resonating cavities, (2) the surface textures of these cavities, (3) the shape of the oral cavity, and (4) the opening or closing of the ends of the nasal and oral cavities.

All vowels are resonant sounds with relative tongue elevation and position represented on the vowel diagram of Figure 7. A number of consonants are also resonant sounds and are sometimes called semi-vowels, vowelized consonants, or liquids because of this characteristic. The resonant consonants are **m, n, ng, w-, y-, l,** and **r.** These consonant sounds usually have a second order designation based on their manner of production to distinguish them from vowel sounds. The **m, n,** and **ng** are designated nasals, since the oral cavity is partially closed off and the nasopharyngeal port is opened to the nasal cavity for their production. The **w-** (as in *went*) and the **y-** (as in *you*) are called ***glides*** since they are of short duration and glide rapidly into the vowel sound which follows. The **l** is called a ***lateral*** since its position with the narrowed tongue point against the alveolar ridge forces emission of voice laterally around both sides of the tongue. The **r** is designated a ***retroflex*** sound because the tongue tip flexes toward the back of the oral cavity.

Another consideration in the manner of production of speech sounds is whether they are voiced or not. Those sounds which include voicing from the larynx are called ***voiced*** sounds. Those without voicing are called ***breath*** sounds, or sometimes unvoiced or voiceless sounds. Occasionally the term "sonant" is applied for voiced sounds and "surd" for voiceless sounds. All vowels and over half of the consonants are voiced sounds.

Phonemes are conventionally categorized in descriptive terms, using the designations of voicing, place of production and manner of production. For example, the **t** is called a breath, lingua-alveolar stop sound; the **v** a voiced, labio-dental fricative; the **l** a voiced, lingua-alveolar, lateral resonant, and the **qu-** a breath, lingua-velar, bilabial affricate. Figure 8 categorizes consonant sounds by their manner and place of production. Recall that the Northampton symbols are arranged on the Yale charts according to place and manner of production for consonants, and by place of tongue arching and lip rounding for vowels.

Manner of Production	Place of Production					
	Labio-Dental	Lingua-Dental	Bi-Labial	Lingua-Velar	Lingua-Alveolar	Lingua-Palatal
Stops			p b	k g	t d	
Fricatives	f v	th¹ th²	wh	h	s z	sh zh
Affricates			qu ←———	qu / x —→x	ch / j	ch / j
Resonants			m w-	ng	l n	r / y-

Figure 8. Consonant sounds ordered by their manner and place of production.

Perceptual Features of Articulation

Another way to view speech production is by the information made available to our auditory, visual, tactile, and kinesthetic senses. To perceive and understand speech requires that the speaker produce acoustic information sufficient for the listener to hear and discriminate among sounds. The study of speech perception, though relevant to teaching speech, is beyond the scope of this book. Chapter III deals with speech perception as it relates to amplification of the acoustic parameters of the speech signal. Additional references of value to the reader are Ladefoged (141) and Malmberg (245). In producing acoustic events through movements of the speech mechanism, the speaker also makes articulatory "gestures" of the lips, tongue, and jaw opening which can be seen by the listener-observer. This information can help the listener in understanding by "speechreading" as he listens. Some of the perceptual features of articulation provide internal feedback information which helps the speaker monitor his speech. Other features may be used by the teacher in her task because they have sensory instructional possibilities.

1. Internal Feedback Information

Pertinent to our purposes is the perceptual information in speech which is made available to the speaker through feedback from his own speech production. This internal feedback information, available through the auditory, tactile, and kinesthetic senses, is essential for the speaker to monitor his own speech production.

Auditory information: As we shall see in some detail in Chapter III, when we talk we produce acoustic signals which have varying features of intensity, frequency, and duration. These features are fed back to the normal speaker by sounds conducted directly through the bones of the skull and by sounds conducted through air into his ear. The severely hearing impaired person is limited to those air conducted sounds which his disordered hearing mechanism can transmit with the assistance of an acoustic amplifier. Even the most severely hearing impaired person seems to get some acoustic information fed back from his own speech with the use of a hearing aid. He may perceive only the presence or absence of sound, a cue to whether he produced voice or not. He may also perceive variations in intensity of sound, a cue to help in monitoring the loudness of his voice and to differentiate among speech sounds.

Speech sounds vary in intensity with a difference of about 28 decibels between the weakest sound and strongest. Strongest are the vowels and diphthongs, and the **w-** and **r-**. Next are the resonant consonants **m, n, ng, y-**, and **l**. In the next weaker group are the voiced fricatives **z, zh, th**, and **v**, the affricate **j**, and the stops **b, d**, and **g**. Then come the voiceless fricatives, affricates, and stops, the **sh, s̩, ch, x, ʠu, p, t**, and **k**. The weakest sounds are the voiceless fricatives **h, f, wh**, and **t̩h**.

With only limited auditory feedback information, the speaker may receive important information about the duration of speech sounds, syllables, and phrases. This information can be of very great help in monitoring the suprasegmental rhythmic features of speech and apparently is very useful for the young deaf child in developing speech rhythm. Frequency feedback information is likely to be very restricted for a severely hearing impaired person. High frequency sounds of consonants are least likely to be available to him. Yet, he may be able to hear some differences in vowel formants which could help monitor his speech.

Tactile information: Another source of speech feedback information is that available to the sense of touch. Tactile information is especially important in helping a hearing impaired person maintain his speech. Tactile features offered by speech production include touching of parts of the speech apparatus, the perception of friction as air flow passes over the tongue, lips, or palate, and the perception of vibration associated with voicing (vibro-tactile). Those sounds offering the most tactile information are the voiceless stops **p** and **t,** where strong contact is made by the lips and by the tongue and alveolar ridge, and the affricate **ch,** which includes the stop of the **t.** In the next group, where there is touching but the force of articulation is decreased, are the **b, d, m, l, n,** and **j.** In the third group are the voiceless fricative consonants marked by strong friction, including **wh, th, f, s̩,** and **sh,** and the affricates **x** and **ʠu.** In the next weaker group are the **k, g,** and **ng,** which have contact in an area which gives little tactile feedback; the **h,** which has its friction between the velum and back of the tongue; and the voiced fricatives $\overset{2}{\text{th}}$, **v, z,** and **zh.** In the weakest group for tactile information are the **w-, y-,** and **r,** the diphthongs, and the vowels.

Kinesthetic information: A third feedback sensation from speech production, kinesthesia, alerts us to the position of parts of the body without seeing them. This sensation is sometimes called "proprioception." The stimulus for kinesthesia is the stretching of muscle fibers as body parts move. Kinesthetic information, like tactile information, is important for monitoring speech. Although there is very little stimulus from movements of the velum and pharynx in closing the nasopharyngeal port, movement of the lower jaw, the lips, and tongue provides considerable kinesthetic sensation. Those speech sounds whose production offer the most kinesthetic information are the lip rounding **aw, oo, w-, wh,** and **qu,** the lip retracted and wide jaw opening **-a-,** and the diphthongs **oi, ou, u-e,** and **o-e,** which offer movement and lip rounding. In the next group are the diphthongs **i-e** and **a-e,** the occasional lip retracted **ee** and the wide jaw opening **a(r),** the $\overset{2}{\text{oo}}$, the voiceless stops **p** and **t,** the fricatives **sh** and **zh,** the affricates **ch** and **j,** and the retroflex **r.** In the third group are the **b, d, y-, m, f, v, l,** and **n.** In the next weaker group are $\overset{1}{\text{th}}$ and $\overset{2}{\text{th}}$, $\overset{1}{\text{s}}$ and **z, k** and **x,** and **-i-** and **-e-.** In the weakest group are the **-u-,** the **h,** the **g,** and the **ng** sounds. Approximate ratings of sensory feedback information for speech sounds are shown in Tables 4 and 5.

	Auditory	Tactile	Kines-thetic		Auditory	Tactile	Kines-thetic
h	1	2	1	**v**	3	2	3
wh	1	3	4	$\overset{2}{\text{th}}$	3	2	2
p	2	5	4	**z**	3	2	2
t	2	5	4	**zh**	3	2	4
k	2	2	2	**j**	3	4	4
f	1	3	3	**m**	4	4	3
th	1	3	2	**n**	4	4	3
s	2	3	2	**ng**	4	2	1
sh	2	3	4	**l**	4	4	3
ch	2	5	4	**r**	5	1	4
w-	5	1	4	**x**	2	3	2
b	3	4	3	**qu**	2	3	5
d	3	4	3	**y-**	4	1	3
g	3	2	1				

5 = *greatest information*

1 = *least information*

Table 4. *Estimated ratings of sensory feedback information for consonants.*

	Auditory	Tactile	Kinesthetic
oo[1]	5	1	5
oo[2]	5	1	4
aw	5	1	5
a(r)	5	1	4
ee	5	1	4
-i-	5	1	2
-e-	5	1	2
-a-	5	1	3
-u-	5	1	1
oi	5	1	5
ou	5	1	5
u-e	5	1	5
a-e	5	1	4
i-e	5	1	4
o-e	5	1	5

5 = greatest information
1 = least information

Table 5.   *Estimated ratings of sensory feedback information for vowels.*

2. Sensory Instructional Possibilities

In addition to the information which makes it possible for the listener to perceive speech and the feedback information which helps the speaker monitor his speech, speech production yields "by-products" which may be exploited by the teacher to provide sensory information in teaching speech.

Visual information: By showing the student his own production in a mirror and by drawing attention to her own model the teacher can present some visible features of speech sounds. These include mouth opening, lip rounding and protrusion, tongue or lips touching the teeth, tongue position inside the teeth, and the degree of jaw opening. Among the most visible speech sounds are the labial and dental consonants, the **m, b, v, f, th[1],** and **th[2]**. Next are the diphthongs which move from one vowel position to another, vowels **aw** and **oo[1],** which involve maximum lip rounding, and consonants **w-, wh, qu, sh, zh, ch,** and **j,** which are also made with some lip rounding. In the third group are the consonants **t, d, n,** and **l,** which offer a view of the tongue just inside the teeth; the **y-, ee,** and **-a-** when they are made with some lip retraction; the **oo[2],** which offers some lip rounding; and the **a(r)** made with wide jaw opening. In the next group the **-i-, -e-,** and **-u-** offer slightly different jaw openings, and the **s[1], z, r,** and **x** offer an obscured view of the front of the elevated tongue. In the least visible group of sounds are the lingua-velar stops **k** and **g,** the **ng,** and the **h,** which takes the shape of the vowel that follows it.

In addition to the ı
products can easily be
ing such simple devices
of air of fricatives or the

Tactile information: T⊦
fingers on the lips, teeth, ⟨
the base of the tongue. Voi
between oral and nasal res⟨
between fricatives and plosi⟨
plosion of breath, can be felt ⟨
between oral and nasal emissi⟨
on the back of the hand.

Speech and Deafness

28

Preceding or following **oo** the point
it is on the hard palate. The dif⟨
koo and **kee** results in pred⟨
Even though both **k** s⟨
has made them sli⟨
k sound in the ⟨
him that it ⟨
Simi⟨
dif⟨

Coarticulation

The influence of adjoining sou⟨ ⟨ines is called coarticulation. This may affect produc⟨ ⟨erceptual features. For example,
the place of production of **k** varies with the vowel sound which precedes it. The
point of elevation of the tongue for the **k** phoneme differs depending on
whether the preceding or following vowel involves front tongue arching or
back tongue arching, illustrated in Figure 9. As the **k** is produced, its point of
contact follows the position of elevation of the tongue for the adjoining vowel.

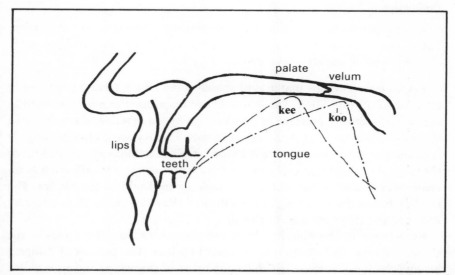

Figure 9. *Relative position of contact of the tongue for implosion of breath
for* **k** *preceding vowels* **ee** *and* **o͝o**.

of contact is the velum, while adjoining **ee**
...erence in place of tongue contact on syllables
...table changes in the acoustic characteristics of **k.**
...nds are recognized as the phoneme **k,** coarticulation
...tly different acoustically. When a listener hears only the
...llable **kee,** the slight acoustic difference may be enough to tell
...as the **ee** sound which followed **k.**
...arly, when the vowel sound is the same in two syllables beginning with
...rent consonants, as in **tee** and **kee,** the relative position of the tongue for
contact on **t** and **k** influences the sound of the following **ee** so that it is slightly
different in each syllable. Note, too, the difference in duration of the vowel **ee**
in the words *eat* and *ease* as a result of the difference in the consonant following and terminating the vowel. The transitional and durational cues present in
coarticulation give the listener important perceptual information about adjoining phonemes.

VOICE

A second major component of speech is voice. Producing voice, like articulating speech sounds, is a function we learn to overlay on structures fundamental to sustaining our bodies.

Production of Voice

Voice is produced by three actions: ***respiration, phonation,*** and ***resonation.***
These occur simultaneously and cooperatively. Together they produce
changes in pitch, quality, and loudness of the voice.

Respiration: The raw material of speech is the breath stream produced in
the process of respiration. The dome-shaped diaphragm moves downward at
the center, reducing pressure in the chest cavity. In reaction, air rushes into
the lungs, filling them as the rib cage expands. The oxygen of the incoming air
is exchanged for carbon dioxide in blood vessels of millions of tiny air sacs of
the lungs. The diaphragm relaxes and the air sacs empty into collecting ***bron-
chial tubes*** leading to paired ***bronchi*** which in turn lead into the ***trachea.*** The
trachea directs the air through the glottis into the pharynx, nasal, or oral cavities, and out either the nose or mouth.

Respiration is accomplished by a complex interaction of muscles of the
thoracic (chest) and abdominal (stomach) cavities. The process of bringing
air into the lungs is called ***inhalation*** and that of evacuating the air is called
exhalation. In normal breathing, the relative duration of inhalation and exhalation is about the same. But when speaking, the duration of exhalation in a

single respiratory cycle is usually about 10 times as long as that of inhalation and may be as much as 50 times as long for practiced speakers. Since no more breath is used in speaking than in regular breathing exhalation, the extended duration of exhalation during speech reflects a remarkable economy in using the breath stream in order to sustain connected speech. This economy, realized by the efficient synergistic functioning of the respiratory muscles, larynx, and articulatory apparatus, apparently is learned.

Phonation: The process of the larynx acting on the exhaled breath stream to create voice is called phonation. The **larynx** (*laryngo-, -laryngeal*) is the complete structure of cartilage and muscles situated atop the trachea, the tube leading to the lungs. The primary purpose of the larynx is to stop food particles from entering the trachea and to expel them with coughing. Also, by closing off the trachea at the larynx, the air in the lungs keeps the thoracic cavity rigid as a help in elimination, childbirth, and heavy lifting.

At the anterior of the larynx, the *thyroid cartilage* forms the "Adam's apple" of the neck. The smaller *cricoid cartilage* rings the bottom of the larynx. Paired *arytenoid cartilages* rest on the cricoid cartilage, providing the paired vocal folds with highly mobile attachments at their posterior ends. The vocal folds, with assistance of laryngeal muscles and the arytenoid cartilages, serve to open and close the trachea at its port called the *glottis.* The laryngeal muscles relax to leave the glottis open, permitting free flow of the breath stream for breathing and for articulation of the breath consonants. These muscles close the glottis by tightly closing the vocal folds but may leave a small chink open between the arytenoid cartilages for the constricted breath stream of whispered speech. They can also close the glottis by lightly approximating the vocal folds so that they are parted by air pressure from the lungs, causing the rhythmic opening and closing of the glottis for phonation.

During phonation, the vocal folds follow this rhythmic cycle: closing of the glottis—increasing of air pressure beneath the glottis—bursting apart of the folds from the air pressure and emission of a puff of breath—closing of the folds again under constant muscle tension and with decreased air pressure. Air pressure beneath the glottis increases and the pattern is repeated. The resulting periodic puffs of breath give the sound of voice. The frequency of puffs of air from closing and opening the glottis determine the *fundamental frequency* of the voice. We can change the fundamental frequency of our voice by a complicated interaction of altering the tension, length, and mass of the vocal folds, accompanied by changing the sub-glottal air pressure.

When there is a considerable increase in the air pressure below the glottis, the vocal folds are forced farther apart during their close-open-close cycle. This increase in vocal fold amplitude is accompanied by an increase in the amount of air emitted and thus an increase in the perceived loudness of the voice. Since the vocal folds are forced farther apart for loud speech, there is also a greater consumption of air.

In addition to voice production, the larynx can contribute an articulated speech-like sound called a *glottal stop.* This sound, which has the IPA symbol / ʔ /, is used in some dialects in place of the medial **t** stop, as in *bottle.*

Resonation: In producing rhythmic closure of the glottis for the fundamental voice frequency, the vocal folds set up secondary vibrations (partials) of their parts which create sounds (overtones) higher than the frequency of the fundamental. These overtones usually are multiples of the fundamental called *harmonics.* If the fundamental voice frequency is 200 cycles per second, or *Hertz* (Hz), the harmonics would be 400 Hz, 600 Hz, 800 Hz, etc. These harmonics differ in their relative intensity, giving a distinctive quality to the sound of the fundamental frequency combined with its harmonics. The harmonics of voice are influenced by cavities of the vocal tract through which voice passes: the trachea, pharynx, oral cavity, and the nasal cavity. These cavities are set into vibration themselves by the flow of vibrating voice passing through them. In vibrating, they reinforce some harmonics of voice more than others, further modifying the overall sound of the voice. This process of modification is called *resonation.* The frequency with which these cavities vibrate and, thus, the harmonics which they emphasize depend on the size, shape, and surface texture of the cavities peculiar to each person. The combination of fundamental voice frequency, overtones of vocal folds, and characteristics of resonating cavities contributes to a complex sound relationship we refer to as *voice quality* or *timbre.*

Most English speech sounds are made primarily with oral voice resonance, that is, with the oral cavity open at the mouth and the velopharyngeal port closing off the nasal cavity at the pharynx. Nasal sounds **m, n,** and **ng** are the exceptions. However, even though the nasal cavity is closed at the pharynx, its resonance contributes to the sound of our voice. Recall how the voice sounds when the nasal cavity is stuffed up with a cold. When the nasopharyngeal port is open for oral resonant sounds, the voice also sounds abnormal with open nasal resonance changing the sound. Nasal resonance is described as *hypernasality* (sometimes called open nasality) when the nasopharyngeal port is abnormally open, and *hyponasality* (sometimes called closed nasality) when the nostrils are blocked making a closed cavity.

Perceptual Features of Voice

Voice produces a combination of auditory, tactile, and kinesthetic information which can be perceived by the listener and speaker.

Auditory information: Phonation produces the fundamental frequency which is heard as the pitch of the voice. The cycles of breath puffs and decreased pressure at the larynx are reflected in the acoustic measure of cycles/second or Hertz (Hz). The fundamental frequency of voice gradually decreases with age, until it rises again in old age. Adult males have a much lower fundamental than adult females. Some typical fundamental voice frequencies are as follows:

Infant hunger wails	512 Hz
Pre-adolescent child	265 Hz
Adult female	225 Hz
Adult male	125 Hz

Fundamental voice frequency for adults can vary from a low of 80 Hz for a male bass singer to over 1,100 Hz for a soprano.

Loudness of the voice, reflected in the physical dimension of intensity, can be altered by increasing the air pressure in the trachea below the glottis. Changes in loudness are used in rhythmic variations of speech, and to overcome background noise, to attract attention, and to adjust to distance. Average speech is about 65 dB sound pressure level (ranging from 60 to 70 dB), measured at about 39 inches (100 cm) from the speaker's mouth. Soft speech is about 45 dB and very loud speech reaches 85 dB. Average speech intensity levels for women are about 3 dB less intense than for men. At about one foot (roughly the distance from the lips to a body-worn hearing aid of the speaker), the average speech level can be 75 dB or greater. Because of a shadowing effect of the head, average speech reaching the ear of the speaker (about 6 inches from the speaker's lips) is not much more intense than that reaching the chest at 12 inches. This shadowing effect of the head is especially pronounced for high frequencies where there is a difference of as much as 7 dB (weaker) for a band of speech 2800 Hz to 4000 Hz reaching the ear, compared to the same speech sounds one foot directly in front of the speaker.

Resonation emphasizes certain overtones of the fundamental voice frequency which give the characteristic formant sounds of vowels. Vowel formants are discussed earlier in this chapter concerning articulation of vowels, and again in Chapter III. Resonation also emphasizes overtones which blend with the fundamental frequency to give perceived voice quality. The normal listener hears his own voice through an almost equal combination of bone conduction and air conduction. He is often very surprised when he hears his voice recorded to know how it sounds to other persons, because his voice sounds different when he hears it only through air conduction.

Tactile information: With voice production, vibration of the vocal folds and of the resonating cavities can be felt in various places on the chest, neck, and head. This vibro-tactile sensation is perceptible both to the speaker through his internal feedback system and to others through their fingertips. The difference between voicing and no voicing, for example, can easily be felt by the presence or absence of vibration. The difference between loud and soft voice can also be perceived by the difference in intensity of vibration, but subtle differences in voice intensity are hard to distinguish through tactile perception. Differences in very high and very low pitched voice can be perceived, but subtle differences in pitch are hard to perceive and may be confused with loud/soft differences. The *difference limen,* the smallest perceivable difference between two stimuli, is quite large for touch. Nasal emission of voice can be perceived by a combination of the place of vibration—especially noticeable on the nose—and generally increased vibration.

Kinesthetic information: Movements of the larynx or within the larynx can give kinesthetic sensations. In changing pitch of the voice, the larynx is raised and lowered giving some sensation of muscle activity. Increasing loudness of voice is often accompanied by increasing tension of the muscles of the larynx. Many of these sensations during speech are at an unconscious level for persons with normal hearing but may be of use to deaf speakers in monitoring their voice.

RHYTHM

Rhythm is often referred to as the prosodic, temporal, or patterned features of speech, or as the "melody" of speech. Speech rhythms are not directly analogous to singing, dancing, or other rhythmic bodily movements, nor are they similar to the common structured rhythms of music. Speech features are rhythmic in that they recur in patterns. Patterns differ from language to language with further differences in dialects and among individuals. Speech rhythm carries meaning, aids understanding, conveys emotional state, and expresses esthetic qualities.

Production of Rhythm

Rhythm features are produced by changes in voice and articulation, and usually by a combination of the two. Changes in intensity, frequency, and duration combine to produce varying "time envelopes" that constitute the fundamental cues for perception of rhythm.

The syllable: In studying articulation we used the phoneme as the basic analytic unit. For speech rhythm, the basic unit is the syllable. Phonemes are not presented to the listener in a haphazard order but occur coarticulated in clusters with consonants bordering vowels. These clusters are called **syllables**. In English the most common syllable cluster is a Consonant-Vowel-Consonant (CVC) combination; less frequently there is a CV or a VC pattern. Such clusters help in our recognition of each phoneme because of the transitional characteristics of consonant-vowel and vowel-consonant junctures which give important perceptual information. During speech, the muscles of the thorax and abdomen controlling exhalation show rapid repetitive pressure fluctuations corresponding to the duration of syllable clusters. The exhalation phase of respiration is marked simultaneously by individual pulses of breath imposed upon the steady exhalation of breath. This muscular action and resulting pulses of breath are the motor basis for syllable production.

Rhythm Features

Relevant to teaching speech are the features of *accent, emphasis, intonation, phrasing,* and *rate. Accent* involves the selection of one syllable to be stressed over other syllables within a word. *Emphasis* is gained by giving increased stress to a word in a phrase. *Intonation* is accomplished by changing pitch from syllable to syllable, rather than from word to word. *Phrasing* of connected speech ignores the boundaries of words and deals with syllable clusters. The *rate* of presenting phonemes to the listener is dependent upon the rate of articulating syllable units.

Accent: Accent is produced primarily by increasing voice intensity and by making stressed syllables longer, but some change in pitch also occurs. It is characteristic of English that every word of more than one syllable has a syllable stressed above the others. For words of several syllables, there may be both a primary accent and a secondary accent. Accent is so common to the English language that its misuse can severely hinder speech intelligibility. Try pronouncing these common words with the accent as indicated: *Ameríca, sylláble, ábove, intéresting, foundatíon.* In order for speech to be intelligible, accent must meet linguistic requirements.

Accent also has an effect on the pronunciation of speech sounds. Unaccented vowels in English lose their original vowel quality and are often pronounced as the -u- phoneme (*above, nation, cobra, telephone, waited*), but with reduced force of articulation reflected by the IPA symbol /ə/. Pronouncing vowels in unaccented syllables with their original vowel quality may actually interfere with intelligibility.

Accent is rarely phonemic in English, that is, it does not change meaning of a word, but it is sometimes used to indicate whether the word is a noun, verb, or adjective. For example, n. *rébel*/v. *rebél;* n. *cómplex*/adj. *compléx;* and adj. *pérfect*/v. *perféct.*

It is impossible to establish hard and fast rules for accent in English words, but some tendencies are helpful. There is a strong tendency for two-syllable words to have their accent on the first syllable. This is especially noticeable in the vocabulary used in the reading books of young children. But the accented syllable usually follows such common prefixes as *a-* (*above*), *be-* (*believe*), *re-* (*report*), *in-* (*intend*), *un-* (*unless*), *ad-* (*admire*), *ex-* (*extent*), and *de-* (*deport*). The accented syllable usually precedes suffixes such as *-tion* (*nation*), *-able* (*desirable*), *-ssion* (*commission*), and *-cious* (*delicious*). The *-ed* ending is rarely accented and the *-ing* ending never is.

Accent is not usually marked in English spelling as it is in some Spanish words, but it may be indicated for instructional purposes with a mark such as / ' / either above the accented syllable or after the accented syllable if syllables are separated.

Emphasis: Emphasis refers to the stressing of a word or words within a phrase. Emphasis, like accent, is produced primarily by a combination of increased intensity and increased duration of syllables within the stressed word, with an accompanying change in voice frequency. It may even be achieved by pauses surrounding words. Emphasis does not have a regular pattern peculiar to the language as accent has, but is used to communicate speaker intent. For example, emphasis may be used to clarify by stressing a single word that reiterates a previous statement ("I mean we absolutely *cannot* finish the work on time."), to contrast with parallel structure ("They walked home but we *drove* home."), and to label something ("We call it a *hydrochronometer*."). Intended meaning determines which word is selected for emphasis. Try speaking the sentence, "My house is five miles down the road," several times and stress each word in turn. Imagine the context in which each of the words might be emphasized.

Emphasis affects pronunciation of speech sounds, too. The preposition *of* is so commonly deemphasized in phrases that its pronunciation /av/ usually becomes /əv/. The phrase "time to go" is commonly pronounced /taɪm tə goʊ/.

Intonation: Intonation refers to variations of pitch in connected speech as a function of time. Intonation patterns are described by the direction of pitch change, the degree of change, and by absolute pitch levels. Absolute levels are extremely hard to specify, since individuals have different fundamental voice frequencies and have different habits of using more or less pitch variation in their speech.

Patterns of intonation are governed both by individual characteristics of talkers and by common usage of the language. We use common intonation patterns to give listeners a secondary level of language information without using additional words. To signal the end of a simple declarative statement, we commonly use a falling pitch on the last word of the statement as in, "I am going home." If there is more to follow after the last word of a phrase, we alert the listener to this by using a very slight drop in pitch or no drop at all, as in, "I am going home and I want you to be there." When we speak of a series of things, each item is given a slightly rising pitch until the last one, which has a falling pitch, as in, "We used the knives, forks, spoons, and plates."

When we ask a question and want the listener to give us a "yes" or "no" answer, we tell him this by using a rising pitch on the last word, as in, "Are you going home?" But when we want him to give us an answer other than "yes" or "no," we frequently end the question with a rising then falling pitch on the last syllables, as in, "Where are you going?" When a question requires a choice of named alternatives, intonation usage places a rising pitch on each alternate, just as it did on a serial statement, and a rising then falling pitch on the last word, as in, "Do you want a knife, fork, spoon, or plate?"

Intonation patterns are not marked in English spelling, but there are a number of ways of designating patterns for teaching purposes. Three common relative pitch levels can be indicated to the student with whole-sentence contour analysis, as in the following (28.14):

Where are you go ing?   I am going home.

A fourth, higher level is reserved for expression of surprise.

My good ness!

Another system uses arrows showing direction of pitch change at certain points in a sentence, either after or above the critical syllables, as in,

Where are you going?   I am going home.

The relative degree of pitch change may be indicated by length of the arrow shaft.

Yet another system marks every syllable for intonation and accent with a dot above unaccented syllables, a line above accented syllables, and a curved line showing rising or falling inflection, as in,

Where are you going?   I am going home.

Phrasing: A speech phrase is a continuous utterance bounded by silent intervals. Phrasing organizes words into groups related to units of thought which help understanding. It has two components—the words linked in speech and the pauses between phrases. Which words get linked and the varying durations of pauses are left to the speaker's judgment, although there are some conventions in the language. Phrasing can help accomplish comparison, as in, "We wanted a red car | but finally bought a yellow one." It can create emphasis, as in, "We must go | now, | before it is too late!" Parenthetical comments, such as, "We must,| I think,| accomplish this tomorrow," are achieved by silent intervals. Note serial items, as in "We used the knives, | forks, | spoons, | and plates."

In addition to these meaning-related conventions, manipulation by the speaker of the number of words in a phrase and the duration of pauses can help the listener understand speech. By increasing the duration of pauses, the speaker takes into account the information absorption rate of his listener for different kinds of content and in different listening environments. The uncertain speaker, who either is not sure how to proceed or is seeking the best possible word to say, uses a pattern of short phrases and frequent long pauses.

Speech phrasing is related to breathing but does not necessarily reflect breathing rhythm. All inhalations during connected speech occur between phrases, that is, during pauses, but inhalation does not always occur with each pause. A speaker may say two, three, or more phrases on the same breath. Figure 10 demonstrates phrasing and inhalation.

With the exception of some punctuation marks, we do not use phrasing symbols in English spelling. But some conventional markings are helpful to indicate word groups, as in "Now is the time, I believe, for all of us to think about changing our attitudes on this matter." Pauses may be indicated by vertical lines using more lines for longer pauses, as in, "Now is the time, | I believe, || for all of us to think about changing our attitudes | on this matter. ||| Now,|| before it is too late."

Rate: Rate refers to the number of syllables uttered per unit of time. It is affected by both stress and phrasing patterns. Stressed syllables are typically longer in duration than unstressed ones. In phrasing, the greater the number of pauses and the greater the duration of each pause, the fewer the units of speech that will be spoken in a period of time. Individuals vary, of course, in the rate at which they talk.

Rate is usually measured by the number of words per minute and the number of syllables per second. Most adults read orally from 160 to 180 words/minute. In connected conversational speech, we average 5 to 5.5 syllables/second (average syllable duration 0.18 seconds) or about 270 words/minute.

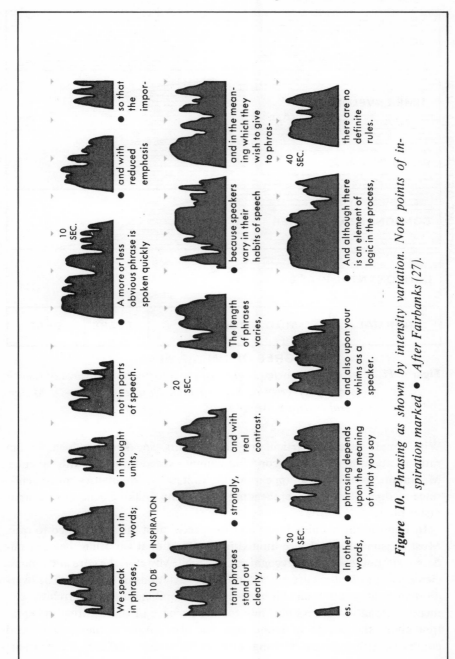

Figure 10. Phrasing as shown by intensity variation. Note points of inspiration marked ● . After Fairbanks (27).

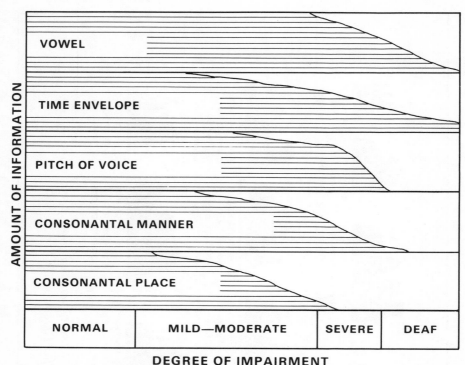

Figure *11. A gross composite estimate of the information features of speech related to severity of hearing loss. Courtesy James D. Miller, Central Institute for the Deaf.*

With simple repetitive articulatory movements, speakers reach maximum rates of about 8 syllables/second but cannot exceed this even with practice. Maximum speaking rate appears to be limited by articulatory movements, since reading silently, comprehending speech, and thinking generally occur at faster rates.

In English, the syllable is the unit of speech most directly related to rate. Most consonant sounds are limited in the durational variation they can undergo without losing their recognizability, while vowels—the core and longest elements of syllables—are not so limited in variations of duration. The overall rhythm of speech is an extremely complex combination of interrelated elements. Intonation occurs not only for the purpose of transmitting information about the nature of a message but also for indicating accents and emphasis, with a generally rising pitch on the stressed syllable. Emphasis is achieved not only by changes of duration and intensity, but also by phrasing, rate, and intonation changes.

Perceptual Features of Speech Rhythm

Since speech rhythm is produced through variations in intensity and frequency of *voice* and in durations of *articulation,* its sensory features will be those described previously under those two headings in this chapter. Speech rhythm, consisting as it does of repeated syllable pulses, gives rise to kinesthetic sensations, probably from the muscles of the thoracic and abdominal areas. The alternating chain of vibrations and pauses set up by syllables may also cause some repetitive tactile sensations in the resonating cavities of the speech apparatus. But it is apparent that these syllable pulses are monitored primarily by auditory sensations. When the auditory system is severely impaired, speech rhythm is drastically affected.

Perception of rhythm may be aided by subtle visual cues. Stressed vowels require positioning of lips and mouth opening for longer times. Movement of the larynx and tensing of laryngeal muscles are manifested in movement at the neck surface. Facial gestures, movement of the head or eyes, frowning, smiling, and facial grimacing are frequently associated with rhythmic patterns.

A gross composite estimate of the information features of speech described above as related to severity of hearing loss is given in Figure 11.

CHAPTER II

Learning and Teaching Speech

S peech is learned. We have noted that speech production is not the primary function of what is commonly and collectively referred to as the speech mechanism. We learn to use parts of the body, developed for more primitive functions, to form the various sounds of speech. Capability for learning to use parts of the body to form sounds and for learning the complex phonetic-linguistic code necessary for meaningful speech is shared by all human beings and is apparently limited to humans. But we are not born "knowing" how to speak. We learn according to the speech patterns around us, growing up learning to speak Chinese, English, or Russian, depending upon where we live. In general, the entire repertory of speech sounds is learned and perfected by age 7.

Learning speech is so universal and apparently so effortless that we take for granted that speech "comes naturally." But when something impedes speech development—when speech is learned poorly or not learned at all—we focus attention on learning to speak and find it to be a complex process. There are numerous requisites for learning speech, and when these are lacking or inadequate, speech will not develop "naturally." Fortunately, we can intervene to improve, revise, restructure, and augment, such as by using other sensory channels in place of or in addition to the auditory. When we do so in order to increase the probability of speech being learned, we are involved in the act of *teaching speech.*

Hearing loss is a major impediment to speech development because it (1) severely restricts reception of speech and (2) reduces ability of the speaker to monitor his own speech. Because both factors are necessary for speech development, a person with severe hearing loss will not develop speech without systematic, comprehensive, and intensive intervention, that is, ***teaching.*** Teaching, in its broad sense, is the act of rational and deliberate intervention in the learning process for the benefit of the student. The charges for the teacher of speech are to understand the process of learning speech and to know how to intervene in order to help the hearing impaired person learn to speak.

For our purposes, we may consider the learning and teaching of speech to involve three primary areas of concern: the ***student*** himself, his ***environment,*** and his ***school program.*** Within each of these areas of concern are significant influences which are important to learning speech. These influences and the overlapping nature of the areas of concern are shown in Figure 12.

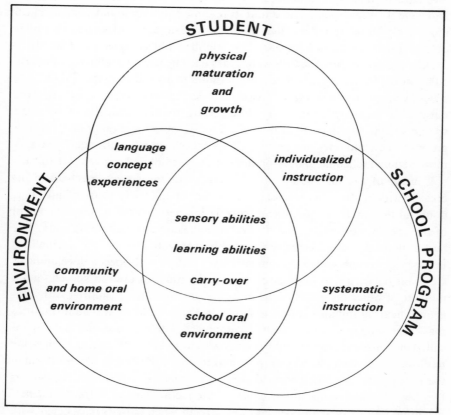

Figure 12. *Areas of concern in learning and teaching speech.*

THE STUDENT

There are a number of characteristics and attributes of the student which affect the learning of speech. Prime among these are the student's physical growth and maturation, and his current and potential sensory capacities and learning abilities.

Physical Growth and Maturation

The young child grows and matures at a fairly predictable rate, with his stages of development reflected in control of his muscular strength and coordination. Schedules of growth and maturation, derived from child development studies, will help the teacher know what skills of motor coordination can be reasonably expected from each child. Speech development depends on motor coordination along with sensory development. The hearing baby babbles speech sounds at random, including sounds which are not those of his language. In a few months he is imitating some babbling sounds, and by age 6 months his babbling reflects the sounds of his language. After one year he is able to form words and increases the number and complexity of words in spoken phrases during the following years until he has a vocabulary of nearly 1,000 words by age 3 years. The jaw continues to grow during the child's early school years, causing increased spaces between his teeth. After age 6 years the baby teeth begin to shed, with missing teeth making articulation of some speech sounds (particularly s) difficult. See Figure 5 for a diagram of dental growth. The child does not perfect all his speech sounds until age 7 years. A more detailed schedule of development in early childhood is given in Table 6.

Control of the fine, small muscle activity of the speech mechanism increases with maturation and experience during the early years of life. It is doubtful that there is a significant correlation between the quality of control of the speech mechanism and of the large skeletal muscles of the body. The best athletes do not necessarily have the best speech. However, abnormalities in physical growth and development may interfere with speech development. Cerebral palsy, which impairs control of the muscles used in speech, and a number of other disorders occur more frequently among children with congenital hearing impairment, as is shown in Table 7. Structural abnormalities may also interfere with speech development. Cleft palate and palatal insufficiency are congenital impairments which make it difficult or impossible to close off the nasopharyngeal port and to direct the breath stream through the oral cavity. Such disorders should be recognized and treated as soon as feasible. Developmental abnormality of the teeth, alveolar ridge, and dental *occlusion* (the fit of the upper and lower teeth when closed) may occur with continual thumb sucking, abnormal swallowing patterns, or habitual mouth

Age (years)	Motor Milestones	Language Milestones
½	Sits using hands for support; unilateral reaching.	Cooing sounds change to babbling by introduction of consonantal sounds.
1	Stands; walks when held by one hand.	Syllabic reduplication; signs of understanding some words; applies some sounds regularly to signify persons or objects, that is, the first words.
1½	Prehension and release fully developed; gait propulsive; creeps downstairs backwards.	Repertoire of 3 to 50 words not joined in phrases; trains of sounds and intonation patterns resembling discourse; good progress in understanding.
2	Runs (with falls); walks stair with one foot forward only.	More than 50 words; two-word phrases most common; more interest in verbal communication; no more babbling.
2½	Jumps with both feet; stands on one foot for one second; builds tower of six cubes.	Every day new words; utterances of three and more words; seems to understand almost everything said to him; still many grammatical deviations.
3	Tiptoes 3 yards; walks stairs with alternating feet; jumps 1 yard.	Vocabulary of some 1,000 words; about 80% intelligibility; grammar of utterances close approximation to colloquial adult; syntactic mistakes fewer in variety, systematic, predictable.
4½	Jumps over rope; hops on one foot; walks on line.	Language well-established; grammatical anomalies restricted either to unusual constructions or to the more literate aspects of discourse.

Table 6. *Correlation of motor and language development. After Lenneberg and Long (241).*

breathing. Health, energy level, and physical stamina, too, are likely to affect a child's ability to learn over sustained periods.

The teacher's responsibility for the physical growth and maturation of the student is generally indirect but nonetheless important. She should be alert to identify, refer, consult, and monitor whenever indicated. In this role the teacher should cooperate with professional workers from other disciplines: developmental psychologists, medical and health personnel, orthodontic and prosthodontic specialists, and speech pathologists. To fulfill her role, the teacher must be aware of their competencies and the contribution each can make to the physical growth and maturation of the learner of speech.

Additional Handicapping Conditions Age	1-5	6-10	11-15	16+
None	61.4	56.2	55.2	59.6
Brain Damage	3.6	3.5	3.5	3.2
Cerebral Palsy	1.6	2.1	2.4	4.2
Epilepsy	0.6	0.6	0.7	0.6
Heart Disorder	2.1	3.2	1.8	0.8
Mental Retardation	2.4	3.9	7.2	8.6
Orthopedic	1.2	0.6	0.7	0.7
Perceptual/Motor	1.5	3.7	3.0	1.0
Emotional/Behavioral	3.2	5.2	5.0	3.7
Severe Visual	2.9	3.9	3.4	2.7
Other	2.2	2.2	2.8	2.7
Blank/Unknown	17.3	14.5	14.1	12.3

Table 7. *Percent of hearing impaired students with specified additional handicapping conditions by age group, United States: 1971-72 school year (124).*

Sensory Abilities

The ability to detect the presence of stimuli, to discriminate differences among them, and to integrate stimuli with previous experience is basic to the learning of speech. The auditory channel is considered primary for speech learning. However, other sensory channels are or may be importantly involved. Along with hearing, we shall consider vision, touch, and kinesthesia. The teacher of speech should be aware of the disorders and remediation for all channels, as well as the contributions of each in learning and maintaining speech.

Vision: Vision is obviously important for utilizing a teacher's speech model and for benefiting from exposure to talkers in the environment. It is also important for providing feedback to the speaker, who watches his listener's face to see whether he is being understood. Consider, for example, the importance that the skilled public speaker attaches to "eye contact." Perhaps because severe hearing impairment is such a conspicuous primary problem for the child with whom we are concerned, mild or moderate impairment of vision may be overlooked. Here is a good illustration of where the alertness of a teacher in identifying a defect may be pertinent to an instructional goal. Surveys among children considered "deaf" have shown that 50% or more have some visual deficiency which can affect their ability to learn, compared to from 20% to

30% of children with normal hearing (197). The visual disability may go unde-
tected and learning difficulties may be attributed to other factors or to hearing impairment, or may be accepted as "natural." Routine visual examinations for all children should begin early and should be continued
periodically to detect defects that may develop with growth or be acquired.
The teacher can also contribute to the student's optimum use of vision by
maintaining a classroom environment with adequate lighting and absence of
glare. Further, she can in her routine activities stress visual awareness and
discrimination of observable differences.

Hearing: As we shall deliberately emphasize throughout this book, the vig-
orous exploitation of residual hearing for the speech development of hearing
impaired children can be of substantial benefit. Note that Chapter III by Dr.
Daniel Ling is devoted exclusively to this topic with emphasis on the fundamental facts of acoustic phonetics that form the basis for teaching procedures. In recognizing the possibilities of residual hearing, the teacher will
need to communicate primarily with audiologists and the student's family,
but in some situations also with otologists, hearing aid dealers, manufac-
turers, and distributors of acoustic amplifier systems. Above all others, the
teacher has the responsibility to see that there is a coordinated and consistent
effort for the student to make the best use of his hearing. Her specific respon-
sibilities include the following:

1.   Maintenance of a good acoustic classroom environment with control
of reverberated sounds from hard, reflective surfaces; control of external
noise sources, such as ventilating ducts, hall noises, building and grounds
maintenance noises; and control of extraneous classroom noises, such as
scraping feet and chairs on hard floor surfaces. The teacher in an "open classroom" should be especially sensitive to the listening stress that such a situation may produce.

2.   Ensuring constancy of hearing aid usage both at home and in school
through the following: by listening to the hearing aids of every child in her
class at least every morning; by having extra hearing aids, spare parts and
batteries available in the school when the student's own aids are not working
properly; by educating the student himself in addition to those who are in
contact with him throughout the day about the use and maintenance of hearing aids; and by having periodic electroacoustic evaluations of the student's
hearing aids to ensure that their gain, frequency responses, power, and distortion characteristics are appropriate.

3.   Ensuring best use of hearing over time by encouraging periodic otologic and audiologic evaluation. This would include examination for possible

acquisition of a conductive component in the hearing loss from cerumen (wax) or middle ear lesions. Parents should be apprised of the need for regular audiologic evaluation, say, once a year. The teacher should report to the audiologist her judgments on the effectiveness of the student's use of his hearing aids in the classroom and confer about recommendations related to the child's hearing or to the performance of his hearing aid. The teacher should be prepared to discuss and apply these recommendations as they bear on her instructional program. The results of audiological tests, particularly audiograms, need to be accessible for handy reference.

4.   *Provision of activities* which give the student opportunity to use amplified sound in the classroom and in his daily routine.

Touch and kinesthesia: Tactile and kinesthetic sensations of speech production may be very important for the speaker with hearing impairment. Experiments in oral stereognosis (the ability to recognize and differentiate the form of objects placed in the mouth) find a correlation between this ability and articulatory skill (95). Whether such tests can yield information about the tactile ability involved in speech production by deaf speakers, or can lead to training and therapeutic procedures, remains for further research. There is yet no evidence that "sense training" which involves recognition of objects by touching with the fingers has any effect on tactile perception of the oral surfaces. The common experience of local anesthesia in dental procedures numbing the tongue and thus affecting speech production demonstrates the role that tactile and kinesthetic senses play in speech production. With sudden loss of hearing in adults and older children, speech production continues in an almost normal manner for some time, even though the auditory monitoring system is absent. This suggests that for the person without hearing loss a system of tactile-kinesthetic speech patterns is developed at an unconscious level, with the auditory system monitoring the output at a more conscious level. In time, without the auditory monitoring system available to determine the accuracy and correctness of speech production, speech becomes less exact and, without special training, eventually deteriorates. It is interesting that the first sound to deteriorate in cases of acquired hearing impairment is s.[1] It has little if any tactile-kinesthetic feedback.

That children have learned speech without the use of hearing is evidence that conscious tactile and kinesthetic sensations can be utilized for learning and maintaining speech. Yet these systems are clearly not as efficient in monitoring as is the auditory system. Persons using primarily tactile-kinesthetic sensations for monitoring speech are not likely to be efficient predictors of the intelligibility of their own speech production (202).

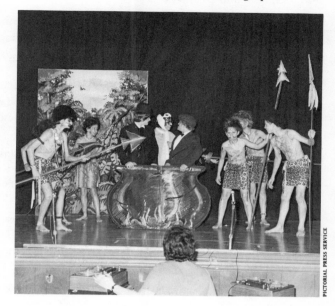

School dramatics encourage speech. A scene from "Around the World in Eighty Days."

PICTORIAL PRESS SERVICE

Learning Abilities

Ability to learn speech depends on more general learning abilities. Pertinent for our purposes are the following learning abilities frequently associated with "information processing": *achievement effort, attention, retention, discrimination and generalization, recognition and recall, formulation,* and *monitoring.*

Achievement effort: Central to the student's achievement effort are his physical condition and his motivation. We earlier described how physical condition affects energy level and tolerance for sustained learning effort. The teacher should recognize that when the student begins to learn speech, his motivations are unique to him, depending upon his experience with previous activities (particularly those in which he has experienced success or failure, pleasure or pain), and upon the pressures of his environment. Motivation can be influenced by the setting of realistic short-term objectives and long-term goals which give the child a chance to succeed at speech tasks, by encouraging identification of the child with peers and adults who use speech effectively, by classroom competition and cooperation, and by tangible rewards. The teacher should motivate speech not as an end in itself, but as a desirable skill relevant to the demands of everyday social experiences and as an opportunity to enrich them. Since motivation is also shaped by a reinforcing environment, the teacher should be aware of the student's proclivities, interests, and activities and offer guidance to the parents to foster motivations that are consistent and satisfying. Hilgard, a noted investigator in learning, suggests the following generalizations about motivation (229):

> A motivated learner acquires what he learns more readily than one who is not motivated. The relevant motives include both general and specific ones—for example, desire to learn, need for achievement (general), desire for a reward, or to avoid a threatened punishment (specific).
>
> Motivation that is too intense (especially pain, fear, or anxiety) may be accompanied by distracting emotional states, so excessive motivation may be less effective than moderate motivation for learning some kinds of tasks, especially those involving difficult discriminations.
>
> Learning under intrinsic motivation is preferable to learning under extrinsic motivation.
>
> Tolerance for failure is best taught through providing a backlog of success that compensates for experienced failure.
>
> Individuals need practice in setting realistic goals for themselves, goals neither so low as to elicit little effort nor so high as to foreordain failure. Realistic goal-setting leads to more satisfactory improvement than unrealistic goal-setting.
>
> The personal history of the individual—for example, his reaction to authority—may hamper or enhance his ability to learn from a given teacher.
>
> Active participation by a learner is preferable to passive reception when learning, for example, from a lecture or a motion picture.
>
> Meaningful materials and meaningful tasks are learned more readily than nonsense materials and more readily than tasks not understood by the learner.
>
> There is no substitute for repetitive practice in the overlearning of skills (for instance, the performance of a concert pianist), or in the memorization of unrelated facts that have to be automatized.
>
> Information about the nature of a good performance, knowledge of one's own mistakes, and knowledge of successful results aid learning.
>
> Transfer to new tasks will be better if, in learning, the learner can discover relationships for himself, and if he has experience during learning of applying the principles within a variety of tasks.
>
> Spaced or distributed recalls are advantageous in fixing material that is to be long retained.

Attention: Essential to processing information about speech is attention through looking, listening, and feeling. The child needs to develop selective or *discriminative attention,* that is, to be able to attend to pertinent (foreground) stimuli while ignoring extraneous (background) stimuli. The time period over which he attends to particular stimuli (attention span) should be progressively extended. Of course, the fundamental aim of the teacher is to develop the child's capacity and desire for self-directed attention.

Retention: The ability to store information is also important. ***Short-term*** retention is involved in both perception and imitation of speech sounds or units of speech, and ***long-term*** retention enables the talker to recall items as needed. To be truly useful, speech needs to be mastered, that is, always subject to immediate and effortless recall. Retention can be developed by relating new information to previous experience, by employing techniques of repetition and review, and by providing an environment in which there is expectancy of recall. Evidence of difficulty in retention may suggest the need for psychological evaluation.

Discrimination and generalization: Learning to talk requires ability to discriminate and to generalize. Discrimination is the determination of critical differences among stimuli; generalization is the determination of critical similarities and includes categorization and classification. Acquisition of fluent speech requires both abilities. While important differences between phonemes (**k** vs. **t,** for example) need to be discriminated, allophonic variations (as for the **k** in **koo** and the **k** in **kee**) need to be generalized as characteristic of a single phoneme.

Recognition and recall: Producing and understanding speech requires calling up bits of information which have been stored in the "memory bank" of the brain. We do this through two means—recognition and recall. To receive and to understand speech requires recognition—the matching of an element with what has been previously stored. To produce speech, other than in imitation, the appropriateness of the needed element is determined by the talker and recalled or retrieved from his memory. It is to be noted that, for production, recognition is generally easier than recall.

Formulation: In addition to recalling sounds required for an intended utterance, the talker needs to formulate or plan how these will be spoken. For example, he must formulate words that convey meaning, linguistic features such as syntactic structure, and intonation patterns that communicate particular intent. In conversation, this process seems to take place in a split second. Relatively little is yet known about formulation or how we can help to develop effective use of this ability, other than to provide practice in varied contexts. For the deaf child, who generally is deliberate in generating spoken language, this poses a formidable challenge. We need to distinguish between a child's ability to produce sounds, or combinations thereof, and his ability to formulate spoken language. The confusion of the two may lead to inappropriate teaching measures.

Monitoring: Monitoring is the process of comparing or matching one's speech to certain standards of speech correctness. For the person without hearing loss, monitoring refers primarily to listening and evaluating his own speech (202). For the person with hearing loss, it also involves in varying degrees tactile and kinesthetic monitoring. The deaf speaker's ability to judge whether he will be understood depends upon how well he can recognize whether his own speech approaches the standard patterns of his culture. He also needs to know from his experience what "errors" in his speech have the highest probability of being a cause of his not being understood and to practice strategies to guide him when a listener asks, "What did you say?" Listener responses also contribute to his monitoring.

THE ENVIRONMENT

The student's total environment is the second major area of concern in learning speech. During his early years, home and community comprise his total environment. Even after he is enrolled in "full-time" school he still spends many more waking hours in this environment than he does in school, not to mention weekends and vacations. Properly and vigorously exploited, the home and community provide valuable opportunities for substantive contributions to growth and development of oral expression. These include language generating experiences, reinforcement of communication through an oral environment, and carry-over of speech behavior from the disciplined situation of the classroom to out-of-school living.

Language Generating Experiences

To speak, the student must have something to say. To have something to say he must have had experiences which lead to ideas that can and need to be expressed in language. It is incumbent upon the teacher to encourage and guide the adults and older children in the child's environment to foster and contrive situations that stimulate spoken language. She should recommend specific activities and suggest how best to take advantage of the significant aspects of experience. Among these are the play activities of the young child, particularly with selected toys. Also valuable are "walking tours" with adults who help discover and examine things of interest, and projects shared with adults which permit the child to participate at his own level. Other children can be a valuable source of experiences that develop concepts to be expressed in language. Properly prepared for and followed up, organized activities can

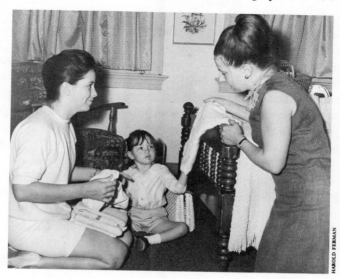

Parent is guided to language learning experiences.

make significant contributions. For the child with hearing impairment, auditory experiences suggest the useful exercise of associating sounds with sources and causes. Parents can make deliberate efforts to expose the child to interesting sounds which can be talked about: the lion at the zoo "roars," the baby "cries," the dog "barks," the door "slams."

Oral Environment

Functional speech is more likely to be learned when practiced in an oral environment where its use is constant, consistent, and meaningful. Essential and salient features of an oral environment are:

1. Speech as the primary means of communication
2. Frequent need to use speech
3. Conventional patterns of speech for the student to perceive
4. Abundant opportunity to use speech
5. Encouragement to use speech.

It is interesting that the absence of even one of these features is often associated with defective speech among hearing children. Consider how indispensable they must be to ensure that the environment has been fully exploited for the speech development of the deaf child.

Carry-over

Carry-over from the classroom to the total milieu of the student implies active collaboration between school and those who are in a position to shape the child's extramural speech behavior. It is certainly more than "homework."

As we have stressed previously, extramural experiences are a rich source for stimulating spoken language. Parents and others should assume the responsibility of communicating them to the school. And, of course, the school needs to do the same for classroom originated language experience. Carry-over, in essence, is best accomplished if it is conceived as a two-way channel of active and informed communication. It means not only that parents visit schools but that teachers visit homes. This sort of communication can provide an atmosphere of supportive attitudes which increase the probability that speech will be used consistently and successfully.

Our advocacy of constructive interchange recognizes the need for rational expectancies of spoken language from the student. Expectancies should neither underestimate nor discourage a child. For one child, even an attempt at speech may be all that can be expected. For another, this may be unacceptable. The layman requires help in what it is reasonable to expect and consequently to encourage. Not to be overlooked is the communication of expectancies to learning contexts in which a child is being "mainstreamed." In a sense, carry-over is the ultimate aim for what goes on in the school. Our experience suggests that the mechanisms and procedures for its accomplishment demand more serious attention than they have been given in the past.

THE SCHOOL PROGRAM

We recall from Figure 12 that a third area of concern is the school program. Wherever the hearing impaired child is educated—whether in a class for hearing children, in a special class in a school system, or in a special school—he requires instruction deliberately designed for learning speech. The design should take into account the quality of the oral environment in the school and systematic programming and organization.

School Oral Environment

No less than the home and community, the school can provide an effective environment that promotes oral communication. The classroom itself can be reinforcing when speech is used as the prominent means of communication in learning language and subject matter. It goes without saying that the lunch period, recess, and school activities of all sorts qualify admirably. From the point of view of motivation for oral expression, they may be crucial in impressing the child with the practical value of his speech skills. Someone in the school should be assigned the responsibility for stimulating awareness and developing procedures to bring this about. In a residential school where the development of speech is taken seriously, the responsibility is to see that this part of the school provides a supportive oral environment. Instructional staff should pursue oral carry-over as vigorously with the dormitory and extramural staff as they do with the parents of day pupils.

What we have said about motivation and practice has special relevance for students in situations where manual communication is emphasized. The purpose of speech may not be clear and thus motivation for speaking may be reduced or absent where the student is encouraged to use a combination of fingerspelling, formal signs of whatever "system," and speech to achieve "total communication." When all the people with whom he communicates daily understand his manual expression, the student is likely to observe that his message can be conveyed by a combination of fingerspelling and signs. *Why then use speech at all?* We believe the justification for students using speech among those who understand manual communication rests on practice for its later use with those who *do not* understand manual communication. Ability to speak widens the circle of situations in which the student can communicate, as illustrated in Figure 1. However, practice on speech in an artificial situation where manual communication is understood is likely to be ineffective compared to situations in which communication *depends* on speech. Experience with learning foreign languages supports this premise. The serious student of speech should experience daily people who do not know manual communication and with whom he needs to communicate. These may include teachers, counselors, resource teachers, and dormitory personnel, as well as the clerks at the neighborhood shops. Fulfilling this requirement of an oral environment is especially important in large residential schools where manual communication prevails.

Systematic Instruction

The speech program of a school should be deliberately and carefully organized, and its central focus should be the provision of systematic instruction. Of course, the development of such a program emphasizes participation by all whose competence, motivation, and responsibility are required for its successful implementation. The prominent features of an organized program include *individualized instruction, methodology,* the discriminating use of *sensory channels and aids,* and *continuity* of programming.

Individualized instruction: Fundamental to an effective systematic program for learning and teaching speech is the determination of the individual needs of each child. This is accomplished by a judicious combination of formal assessment of speech skills and continuing critical observation of speech behavior in all contexts. The results of assessment and observation should be the basis for decisions pertaining to placement, instructional procedures, and current and projected expectancies. The integration of an analysis of needs with a plan for action based on them should constitute the ***child's individual speech program*** for a conveniently designated period of time, probably an academic year. We are aware of the difficulty of achieving individualized instruction in conventional settings but our experience dictates that this is essential. Comfortable compromises on this point can negate the best of intentions to cultivate oral performance. Furthermore, in planning for individuals the teacher should not be constrained by the requirements of appealingly organized plans that address themselves to graded levels of speech.

Methodology: There are numerous "methods" advocated for teaching speech, as we shall see in Chapters V and VI. What merits the designation "method" is an open question. In our view a method consists of the selection of techniques consistent with general strategies of teaching speech. Fundamental to a method is a carefully determined rationale that reflects a working understanding of the array of options whose value has been demonstrated by experience. The teacher needs to know why she does what she does. Hit and miss procedures are to be avoided.

An example of generating methodology is in selecting techniques for correcting errors. Suppose a primary age student, intending to say the word *by,* has said a word that sounds like *pie,* substituting **p** for **b**. A number of techniques are at hand to "correct" the error. But which to choose? The teacher knows that speech instruction should support practice that strengthens maintenance of a skill of which the child is judged to be capable. This suggests to the teacher that she choose a strategy to reinforce long-term memory for speech production. She should give the student an opportunity to recall the correct (or his best) production, rather than identifying the error by presenting a model for imitation of the correct sound. She knows that simple imitation is not the technique of choice to develop the child's ability to decide what is required to accomplish intelligibility and then to retrieve the appropriate sound from his stored repertory.

With this in mind, in order to signal an error, she may begin by telling the student she did not understand all of his last sentence. This technique gives the student maximum opportunity to appeal to his catalogue of ***internalized error probabilities applicable to the particular utterance.*** This may enable him to make the correct sound in the same context in which it was originally in error. If he repeats the sentence with the same error, the teacher may elect to point the student in the direction of the error, but without identifying it, by writing the word in which it is contained. Or she may give him a more explicit clue, underlining the incorrect sound. The student now has the opportunity to concentrate on what he has learned about the manner and place of production of **b** and such error as he may frequently make. If the student still does not make the **b** sound correctly in the word, the teacher may go a step further and write the letter "p" immediately above the letter "b" and then cross out the letter "p". This lets the student know the nature of his error. Now he may think through the differences in producing the **p** and **b** sounds and attempt the correct production.

Each technique the teacher has selected is consistent with her strategy of giving the student opportunity to recall what he had previously learned. She began with a technique which required considerable identification, analysis, and recall by the student, and when he was unable to correct himself, she gave him progressively more information. The next time he makes the error, he may need less help in correcting it. Sustained experience of this sort should contribute to the skill and confidence with which he responds to situations in which he is not immediately understood.

It is well here, as we consider the strategy of methodology, to remind ourselves of our statement in the Introduction of our intent to "enhance the teacher's power to analyze the task of speech instruction." A useful guide to accomplish this is to specify essential components of the act of teaching as they apply to speech. In a sense, they constitute the basis for a "lesson plan"! These components are (28.3):

1. Orientation
2. Stimulation for production
3. Reinforcement by reward
4. Repetition
5. Running evaluation.

1. Orientation is the frame of reference in which the teaching act takes place. It includes development of the child's individual speech program and sensitivity to the educational context in which speech will be taught—as a separate act, associated with other modes of communication, or concurrent with other instruction. It also involves carefully thought-out goals and procedures to stimulate a constructive motivational set for learning. Obviously, attention to the physical elements of the environment such as lighting, acoustics, esthetic decor, and arrangement of equipment is required.

2. Stimulation for production suggests a progression that derives from the principle that "natural" speech development is the preferred, but frequently not the sufficient, basis for speech instruction. Hence, the progression represents a gradient of decreasing naturalness or increasing contrivance: reinforcement of correct spontaneous production, planned stimulation with a direct attempt at production by the student, awareness of error as illustrated above, deliberate elicitation of imitation of the teacher's speech pattern, demonstration of the place and/or manner of production of speech sounds, and, finally, manipulation of the student's speech mechanism.

3.   Reinforcement by extrinsic *reward* of whatever timing, frequency, or nature (gold star, teacher praise) implies the need for the teacher to convey to the student the kind of speech behavior which elicits reward. Effective teachers do this intuitively. Yet the analysis requires attention to reinforcement and certainly to our ultimate aim that speech is its own reward. The student should come to recognize that his ability to communicate by speech expands the compass of his entire existence.

4.   Repetition contributes importantly to the achievement of unconscious spontaneous production of speech, that is, to its mastery. This may involve a range from specifically targeted speech drills to elicited repetition in real-life situations. Whatever the item or context—whether simple consonant-vowel-consonant nonsense syllables, coarticulated clusters, or spontaneous utterances originated by the talker—the opportunity for purposeful repetition needs to be evaluated and acted upon.

The construction of speech drills needs to be based on certain essential principles. These are: (1) The drill should have a clearly stated purpose such as learning something new, or fixing or maintaining what has been learned. It should not be a useless "going through the motions." (2) When possible the child should know the reason for the drill. (3) Phonetic permutations should be adequately sampled. For example, a vowel drill should have stops and fricatives following the vowel; a consonant drill should combine with samples from all vowel classes. (4) The timing of a drill should be determined by the child's abilities at a given stage in his development. A child may be able to give a final **t** but may not be ready to generalize to production of final **t** in words ending in *-ed* as in *looked.* Complicated clusters should be introduced gradually. (5) The child should get reasonably frequent feedback about his performance with care taken to avoid reinforcement of inappropriate production.

5.   Running evaluation refers to a kind of daily inventory of a child's performance that may influence speech work to be modified and adapted both immediately and cumulatively to shape longer-range strategies.

Discriminating use of sensory channels and aids: Knowledge of the sensory capabilities of a child should obviously lead to the specification of their optimum use. Optimum use requires *discriminating* use by the teacher of sensory channels and aids. How often we observe indiscriminate use! Consider the teacher as a frequent "sensory aid" who places the hand of a child on her face presumably to transmit information about a sound over the child's tactile channel. Some teachers whom we have observed usually place the hand over the same area of the face without regard to such factors as what cues she wishes to transmit (loudness, manner, or what?), the discriminability of the item over the tactile channel, the quality of the signal, irrelevant and obfuscating information in the signal (muscle tension), and facilitation or inhibition of the message when combined simultaneously with its audibility and visibility.

For example, consider the possibility of transmitting the distinction between **z** and **zh** over the tactile channel. Place the fingertips on the neck muscle (the sterno-cleido-mastoideus) just below the mastoid process of the temporal bone. Here, both sounds are sensed, but the vibro-tactile sensation for **zh** seems to cover a larger area than for **z.** If the fingertips are not directed to this area, the distinction is not communicated. Teachers should practice these possibilities on themselves. If possible, they should do it with noise in their ears to eliminate acoustic cues.

On the other hand, pragmatic use of channel and aid is indispensable to systematic instruction. The range of possibilities for generating speech or speech related signals appropriate to the child's sensory capabilities needs to be carefully considered, along with the *mode* to be used over a particular channel; whether, for example, over the visual channel a signal should be lipread, fingerspelled, written, or diagrammed. It is among these that the teacher needs to make discriminating choices for a particular purpose.

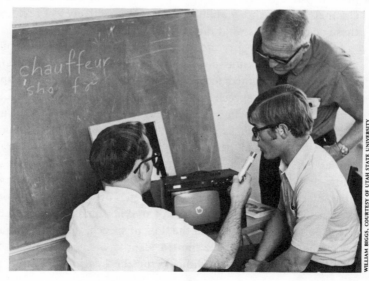

**A visual
sensory aid.**

WILLIAM BIGGS, COURTESY OF UTAH STATE UNIVERSITY

Implicit in these comments is the view that the primary sensory aid is the teacher. In the classroom she is an ever-present interacting aid, shaping her own immediate input to the child in response to his speech behavior. She decides when and whether to intervene in order to reinforce, correct, or improve speech, not to mention her important role in its development. In doing so, she has to make a choice of channel and mode to communicate to the child. Should she use his ears, his eyes, his skin, or some combination of these? Should she speak louder? Should she show the child the placement of her tongue? Should she have him feel the stream of air characteristic of a fricative consonant? Her decision will depend on the particular circumstances, based, of course, on her knowledge about the child as previously delineated in this chapter. What we are stressing here is that she exploit the possibilities inherent in her own person in communicating information about speech.

The teacher is uniquely capable of presenting to the child the kinds of isomorphic sensory cues necessary for his own monitoring. These do not require transformation of the signal. For example, an "S" Meter, on the face of which a needle is directed toward a target point when a child produces a proper s̓, requires the child to transform this visual information to properly shape his tongue to produce the s̓. This is not his natural feedback mechanism. An ideal instrument would present him with a stream of air flowing through a central aperture shaped by the tongue. A teacher can produce this stream of air herself. Along these lines, we have suggested in Chapter IV the "sensory instructional possibilities" of the various phonemes. Tables 8 and 9 present our estimates of the ordering of these possibilities with respect to channel. The teacher's ability to interact effectively in "real time" to exploit these possibilities is what makes her the primary sensory aid.

Nevertheless, sensory aids—considered from the conventional standpoint as supplements but not substitutes for the teacher—can be useful. Some sensory aids are designed to extract and transmit features of speech that are likely to facilitate speech perception and hence speech production. Selective amplification in hearing aids (elaborated in Chapter III), visual displays of pitch dynamics such as glides, and transmission of nasal/non-nasal, voice/voiceless features to stimulators on the skin illustrate the range of possibilities that have attracted the attention of engineers and investigators. We know, too, that speech is a signal whose characteristics change rapidly in time. The rapidly changing perceptual cues of speech place upon the auditory system the essential requirement of making quick decisions about what has been spoken. As he listens to the flow of speech, the listener must be quick to select the cues that enable him to identify a sound as being different from all other sounds. This is difficult for the hearing impaired person to do.

	Visual	Tactile		Visual	Tactile
h	1	4	v₂ / th	5 / 4	4 / 3
wh	4	5	z	1	2
p	5	5	zh	2	4
t	3	4	j	2	1
k	1	3	m	5	5
f₁	5	4	n	3	5
th₁	4	4	ng	1	5
s₁	1	2	l	3	2
sh	2	3	r	2	2
ch	2	4	x	1	3
w-	4	5	qu	4	4
b	5	4	y-	2	4
d	3	4			
g	1				

5 = greatest possibilities
1 = least possibilities

Table 8. Estimated ratings of sensory instructional possibilities for consonants.

	Visual	Tactile
oo¹	3	4
oo²	2	5
aw	3	5
a(r)	2	5
ee	2	4
-i-	1	4
-e-	1	4
-a-	2	5
-u-	1	5
oi	5	5
ou	4	5
u-e	5	4
a-e	3	4
i-e	3	4
o-e	4	5

5 = greatest possibilities
1 = least possibilities

Table 9. Estimated ratings of sensory instructional possibilities for vowels.

Primary Factors of Speech	The Teacher	Common Classroom Devices	Sample Electronic Equipment*
VOICE			
Loudness	Intensity of acoustic signal (A)	Balloon on teacher/child face (T)	Light activated by microphone (V)
	Intensity of vibration on skin (T)	Musical instruments (A)(T)	Tactual vocoder (T)
Pitch	Frequency of vibration on skin (T)	Musical instruments (A)(T)	Pitch meter or indicator (V)
	Vertical movement of larynx (T)(V)		
Nasal / Non-Nasal	Place of vibration on skin (T)		Nasal indicator (V)
Quality	Display of muscle tension and relaxation (T)(V)		
ARTICULATION			
Manner of Production			
Voicing	Vibration on skin (T)		Tactual vocoder (T)
Breath	Breath on skin (T)		
Force of Articulation	Exaggerated force (V)(T)	Feather, flame, paperstrip (V)	
Place of Articulation	Model as static display (V)	Diagram, model, mirror (V)	Vowel indicator (Oscilloscope)(V)
	Model exaggeration (V)		Spectrograph (V)

(continued)

Acoustic Features Intensity Frequency Duration Dynamics of Co-articulation	Gesture (duration) (V) Model as slow motion (V) Manipulate speech mechanism (K)	Written symbol codes (V)	"S" meter (V) Spectrograph (V)
RHYTHM Rate	Model (A) Gesture (V)		
Stress (accent, emphasis)	Model (A)(V)(T) Pressure on hand (T)	Written symbol codes (V) Musical instrument (A)(T)	Light activated by microphone (V) Pitch level meter (V) VU meter
Intonation	Model	Written symbol codes (V) Musical instrument (A)	
Phrasing		Written symbol codes (V) Musical instrument rhythm (A)(T)	

Table 10. Digest of sensory aids applied to the *primary factors of speech.* *(A)* = *Auditory,* *(V)* = *Visual,* *(T)* = *Tactile,* *(K)* = *Kinesthetic Senses.*

(*The Hearing Aid, which applies to all features of speech, is treated in Chapter III.)

Speech is simply too fast for him. The confusion in the dynamics of speech may be somewhat ameliorated by a static visual display that "freezes" a feature to be communicated and then reproduced. An example of this is a display of pitch change (frequently a line changing in horizontal and vertical dimensions) which can be contemplated by the student and serve as a target for his own production.

Sensory aids can add to the convenience, frequency, and accessibility of speech experience not easily provided by the teacher. By speaking louder, of course, she can amplify sound—which is what the most popular sensory aid, a hearing aid, does. But she is not likely to be able to do this over a sustained period of time. Hearing aids do not get tired and they can and should be with the user all the time. Also helpful as sensory aids are models, diagrams, and films that display pertinent aspects of the speech act. A transparent model of the head with moving parts that can be manipulated makes visible some movements and structures that are hidden, like the raising and lowering of the velum. Diagrams effectively demonstrate the arching of the tongue, and ingenious films illustrate tongue movement and laryngeal action.

Sensory aids can provide vehicles for self-instruction, particularly in their role as "error detectors." They can be imaginatively designed to appeal to children's interests and to motivate practice. Children have been observed to be intrigued by banks of bright colored lights used to signal loudness or pitch change. Here is an opportunity for enthusiastic proponents of "behavior modification" to develop suitably programmed "rewards" for appropriate speech production. Table 10 contains a digest of the application to the primary factors influencing the intelligibility of speech of an array of sensory aids and the sensory channels to which they apply. Increasing classroom experience and ongoing research promise an augmented and progressively refined stock of aids.

A teacher's discriminating use of sensory aids—whether of her own person, common classroom devices, or elegant electronic instruments—demands of the teacher a continuing concern for their value. Does the aid deliver what is intended? Will something simpler do just as well? Does the result justify the expenditure of time, energy, and money? Will apparent initial motivation wear off? Is there evidence that it carries over to extramural speech situations? It is important to note that such "hard" evidence as exists for the value of engineered visual and tactile sensory aids is based on short-term data from laboratory contexts. It is incumbent upon investigators to carry on evaluations in the classroom and in everyday speech situations. Here is a splendid opportunity for teachers and investigators to collaborate effectively in pursuit of a common goal. As much as anything, the deliberations of recent conferences on speech analyzing aids, sensory training aids, and sensory capabilities of hearing impaired children point emphatically to this need (52, 63, 191).

Continuity of program: Continuity implies a sequence of empirically accumulated children's individual speech programs—each building on the previous one and directed to the ultimate goal of intelligible speech. While each teacher develops an annual program, supervisors should ensure that there is continuing progress in gaining speech skills over a number of years. Without school-wide coordination, the disjointed and discontinuous efforts of individual teachers—some of whom may be transient members of a staff—can contribute to confusion, insecurity, and negativism toward speech. Illustrative of what frequently characterizes discontinuity is variation in systems of orthography, in appeal to devices such as color codes and particular sensory aids, and in convictions of the teacher as expressed in the recognition of the features of an oral environment previously listed.

Chapter III

Amplification for Speech

Daniel Ling

There would be no need to teach speech to hearing impaired children if hearing aids compensated fully for all types and degrees of hearing loss. Like normally-hearing children they would perceive the speech of others, monitor the speech they themselves produce, and acquire speech and language "naturally." Some hearing impaired children can acquire normal speech communication skills through the use of hearing aids. But the greater the hearing loss, the less chance there is of completely natural speech acquisition; and the later the beginning of instruction, the greater becomes the need for skilled speech teaching. Total deafness is rare, and hearing—however limited—is the most effective modality for teaching most aspects of speech. Hearing aids are therefore useful tools for the teacher of deaf children in developing speech.

HEARING AIDS

There are many makes and types of hearing aids. The most common is the **personal aid** which may be worn on the body or on the head, the latter either behind the ear or incorporated in eyeglasses. Most of these aids contain a coil which can be used when listening to the telephone or to sound relayed through an **induction loop**. Hearing aid systems which employ **radio frequencies** to transmit sound from the teacher to the pupil are more and more frequently used in special schools and classes for the hearing impaired. In some such systems the children wear special **FM hearing aids;** in others they can use their

64

own personal aids. Many schools are also equipped with conventional **group hearing aids** (wired systems), and some teachers or clinicians use individual (table model) speech training aids. Because wired or table model systems usually employ high quality components and need not be miniaturized, they are generally capable of reproducing sound with higher fidelity than the smaller personal aids. All types of hearing aids mentioned above have one thing in common: they provide some degree of amplification, or **gain**.

Gain

The gain of the hearing aid, measured in **decibels** (dB), is defined either as the amount the sound pressure level is increased at 1000 Hertz (Hz) or as the average increase of intensity over the three frequencies 500, 1000, and 2000 Hz. Hearing aids are usually fitted with a volume control to vary gain over a given range. How much gain is required to amplify speech sounds so that they are audible to a hearing impaired child? This depends on two things: the intensity of the speech reaching the aid and the child's hearing level. If a speech sound has to have a sound pressure level of 110 dB to be clearly audible to a deaf child, and that sound reaches the microphone of his hearing aid at 60 dB, then the aid must have a gain of 110 − 60 = 50 dB to provide adequate output. In general, INPUT + GAIN = OUTPUT. Thus, one can also provide an output of 110 dB by using a stronger voice and less gain. For example, speech at 80 dB and a gain of only 30 dB would also yield an output of 110 dB. Amplifiers in which output increases in direct proportion to input are said to have **linear gain**. Linear gain can operate only over a certain range because all amplifiers have an upper limit of output power which cannot be exceeded. If gain plus input add to more than this ceiling, the amplifier becomes overloaded and output becomes distorted.

Providing a constant input to a hearing aid can be seen as a difficult task. Voice levels vary considerably from one speaker to another. Each speaker uses different voice levels at different times to stress a particular point, to reflect an emotional state, or to be heard above background noise. In addition, the distance between speaker and listener profoundly affects the intensity of speech. When distance is doubled, the sound pressure level of speech under non-reflecting conditions drops by 6 dB. To the normal listener, variations in speech level make little difference to either its audibility or intelligibility because the **dynamic range** over which the normal ear functions is wide.

We may think of the dynamic range as being a region bounded by the quietest sound which can be heard at one end of the scale and the loudest sound which can be tolerated at the other. The dynamic range over which many hearing impaired children function, however, is quite restricted. Speech sounds which may be audible when the speaker is a few inches from the microphone may be inaudible when the distance is increased to a few feet. The problem cannot be overcome simply by providing more powerful hearing aids because hearing impaired listeners may tolerate loud sounds less well than do normal listeners. If hearing aids with linear gain characteristics are used in teaching speech to children whose dynamic range of hearing is very restricted, then speech input level must be carefully monitored and maintained at a fairly constant intensity. Accordingly, many wired systems incorporate a VU meter which allows the teacher to monitor the intensity of her voice.

To permit output levels to remain fairly stable when input levels fluctuate widely, and to ensure that output does not become uncomfortably loud, some amplifiers have circuits which provide some form of *automatic gain control* (AGC). Linear compression and curvilinear compression are both used for this purpose. *Linear compression* operates so that speech is compressed by a constant amount over a wide dynamic range. Thus, beyond a given point an increase in input increases the output by a fixed ratio of less than one. In other words, gain is decreased by a constant amount as input is increased. This contrasts with *curvilinear* compression, which operates in a linear way at low input levels but increasingly reduces the amount by which sound is amplified beyond successively higher input levels.

Peak clipping is also used to limit output. As its name suggests, it prevents output from exceeding a certain selected level simply by clipping off the peaks of syllables which are too intense. In quiet, this method detracts little from intelligibility, but in certain types of noise, intelligibility is greatly reduced. The use of hearing aids with some form of automatic output limiting is now quite common, but the effects of the different types of circuitry on speech discrimination skills have not yet been adequately studied.

Input, Gain, and Noise

Noise, defined as unwanted sound, occurs in most real-life situations. Sometimes its level is so high that it interferes with our understanding of speech. People with sensorineural hearing loss respond to speech in noise as if the noise level were substantially greater than it is. To use the child's defective hearing effectively in teaching him to speak we must, therefore, ensure that noise does not interfere with our work unnecessarily. Indeed, a severely hearing impaired child is likely to learn to discriminate and produce speech effectively only under good acoustic conditions.

As we have seen in Chapter I, vowel sounds like **aw** may be 30 or 40 dB louder than soft unvoiced consonants like **f**. The dynamic range of speech, therefore, is 30 to 40 dB. To ensure that a child hears all speech sounds under the best conditions, a **signal/noise** ratio (S/N), that is, speech level minus noise level, of 30 dB is desirable. If the ambient noise level of the room in which you wish to teach is 50 dB in the speech frequency range, then your loudest speech sounds would have to be at 80 dB if the quietest ones were to be stronger than the ambient noise. This is possible under only two conditions: first, if the microphone of the aid is close to the teacher, or second, if she shouts from a greater distance. But shouting is not only a strain on the speaker; it has major disadvantages. The louder one talks, the greater the dynamic range of one's speech becomes. To verify this, try saying the words *farm* or *four* both quietly and loudly. You will hear that the initial **f** changes very little in amplitude in comparison with the phonemes that follow. Thus, quiet speech near the microphone is clearer than loud speech at a distance, not only because it is less distorted or reverberant, but because its dynamic range is smaller. In sort, the possibility that unvoiced consonants can be heard in quiet speech is increased.

As mentioned earlier, sound pressure, in the absence of reflection, drops by 6 dB with the doubling of distance. This relation between distance and sound pressure level is illustrated in Figure 13. This figure, in which the ambient noise level is depicted as 50 dB over the speech range, shows that speech reaching a level of 80 dB at 3 inches from the lips drops to only 50 dB, the ambient noise level, at 8 feet. At 3 inches the S/N ratio is 30 dB; at 8 feet it is zero. In real life, fortunately, conditions are not usually as depicted in Figure 13. Rooms are usually reverberant and most of the energy in ambient noise tends to be lower in frequency than speech.

Figure 13 shows that input of everyday speech varies inversely with distance. To obtain desired output levels (INPUT + GAIN = OUTPUT), one must either control input level or gain or both. In most teaching situations control over distance from the microphone is fairly easily achieved since either wired systems or induction loops can be used. With the exclusive use of personal aids, a position close to the microphone of the amplifying system which gives optimum, noise-free, high intensity input is hard to attain.

Speech can, of course, be discriminated in certain types of noise. But as the noise becomes more continuous, as the components of the noise become more varied, and as the S/N ratio becomes poorer, discrimination tends to become worse. Although the research demonstrating this has been on normally-hearing listeners, it is reasonable to generalize such findings to hearing impaired adults and children with the following caveats: first, noise more drastically interferes with speech perception in the hearing impaired and, second, even more drastic interference might be expected in the case of hearing impaired children who have not yet acquired normal language and all the perceptual advantages that the possession of high-level language skills lend to speech discrimination.

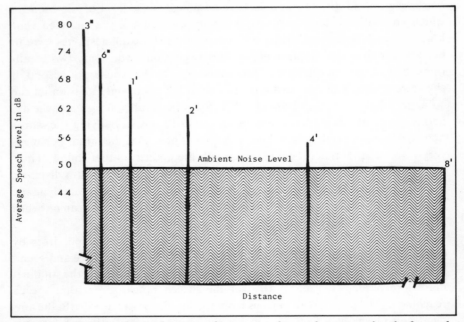

Figure 13. *The relation between distance and sound pressure level of speech in a non-reverberant room with an ambient noise level of 50 dB.*

Frequency Range

The effects of frequency range on speech and music are well known. Both come across much more naturally on high fidelity equipment than through small radios. This is because small radios, like the telephone and most personal hearing aids, reproduce frequencies only from about 300 to 3000 Hz, a range which excludes much of both speech and music. In contrast, high quality group or speech training aids driving high quality earphones encompass the range 70 to 7000 Hz.

Components of speech are as low as 100 Hz and range to above 8000 Hz. The lowest sounds are the voice *fundamental frequency.* A male speaker may have a lower voice than a female speaker, yet if both say the same sentence, the linguistic elements such as phonemes are heard as being much the same even though the nonlinguistic elements or variants which carry information on age, sex, and emotional state are recognized as being distinctly different. Thus speech contains *invariant cues*—those that permit the identification of the speech sounds themselves, and *variant cues*—those relating to the speaker and to the *suprasegmental* aspects of speech such as stress and intonation. For children who have little or no hearing above 1000 Hz, the use of hearing aids with a frequency range extending down to 100 Hz rather than to 300 Hz has been shown to be advantageous in perceiving and producing the variant and suprasegmental aspects of speech. These aspects are important in everyday communication and are frequently abnormally produced or missing in the otherwise-good speech of the orally educated deaf child. The full use of hearing aids to exploit residual hearing appears to be essential for the adequate development of these aspects of speech.

What of the so-called invariant cues which allow us to identify actual speech sounds? In fact, as pointed out in Chapter I, they are far from constant. In running speech they vary in relation to the context in which they are spoken. The way the articulators have to move in order to make one sound after another in sequential patterns influences the frequency, intensity, and duration of each phoneme in an utterance.

The vowel sounds are each characterized by two or three formants, or peaks of energy, which result when the cavities of the vocal tract resonate. For each vowel, the tongue and lips assume a different position and thus create the cavities and apertures which determine the frequency of each vowel formant. These formants tend to be lower for male than for female and child speakers, although their relative positions on a logarithmic frequency scale are similar. Most of the vowels of English are present in the sentence, "Who would know more of art must learn and then take his ease." *Spectrograms* of this sentence spoken by the writer are shown in Figure 14. In spectrograms the frequency of the sounds is represented on the vertical axis. In the example given in Figure 14, the frequency range is from 80 to 4000 Hz. Duration is read along the horizontal axis and each spectrogram shown represents almost 2.0 seconds of speech. Intensity is represented by the degree of shading. Strong components are dark, weaker components lighter. The dark bars near the bottom of the spectrograms are known as voicing bars and represent the fundamental (F_0) of the writer's voice, which is in the range of 90 to 120 Hz. The first formant (F_1) is the dark bar just above the F_0 and the second formant (F_2) is the third dark bar. The vowels in the sentence are seen to be arranged so that F_2 increases in frequency as the sentence is spoken. It will become evident why this sentence provides very useful reference material for the teacher.

The spectrograms confirm that each vowel has its own characteristic formants, quite unlike those of other vowels. Now, imagine a hearing aid which cuts out all sounds below 500 Hz. By placing a ruler horizontally across the spectrograms, just about halfway between the base line and 1000 Hz, it can be seen that quite a lot of information is lost. The low frequency components of the nasal sounds disappear, the formant structure of the first word is destroyed, and the vowel **oo** weakened, perhaps to the point where it becomes inaudible to a severely hearing impaired child. Now place the ruler so that sounds below 1000 Hz can be isolated. The sounds of speech which are available to a child with hearing up to this frequency are seen to be the back and mid vowels, that is, the vowels in the first half of the sentence and most of the voiced consonants. Thus even children with limited hearing can be seen to have a considerable amount of auditory information on speech available to them. The speech needs to be amplified, but it falls within the frequency range readily reproduced through modern aids.

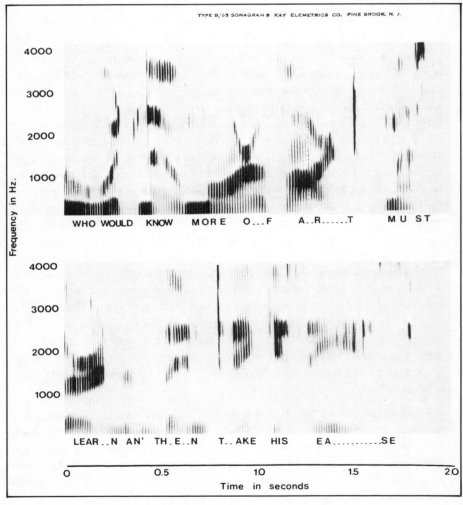

Figure 14. Spectrogram of a sentence.

The art of teaching has been defined as working from the known to the unknown, from the easy to the difficult. In teaching speech to hearing impaired children we can add, "and working from the audible to the inaudible." For example, if voice/voiceless distinctions are hard for a child with residual hearing to discriminate and reproduce, one should work on obtaining the distinction first using consonants together with back vowels. Whether a consonant is heard as voiced or voiceless partly depends on whether there is a lag between the release of the consonant and the onset of voice. A lag in voice onset time, which is an important acoustic cue signaling a voiceless consonant, can be seen on the spectrograms in Figure 14 in the words *who, take, then,* and *his.* In these words, F_2 clearly precedes the voicing bar. Now the second formants of all back vowels are audible to a child with residual hearing below 1000 Hz, whereas those of front vowels (the last words in the sentence) are not. If the voice/voiceless distinction, characteristic of the cognate pair **p–b,** is learned in the context of back vowels, it may be generalized to other cognate pairs, **t–d,** and **k–g,** and to their use with mid and front vowels.

The upper end of the frequency range of most personal hearing aids has until recently rarely exceeded 3000 to 3500 Hz, a limitation imposed by the difficulty of engineering high quality miniature microphones and receivers. There may be a trading relation between output and frequency range. Some aids with condenser microphones do have a frequency range up to 5000 Hz. To examine the potential advantage of this wider range for those who have hearing above 3000 Hz, place a ruler horizontally across the spectrograms of Figure 14 to occlude components above 3000 Hz. While the majority of vowels are unaffected, unvoiced consonants are either attenuated or excluded by such filtering. Take for example the **sh** and **s** sounds in Figure 15. The former loses a great deal of its energy, the latter is nearly completely destroyed. The characteristic frequencies of **s** lie in the range 3500 to 8000 Hz. If the frequency range of the hearing aid is from 250 to 3000 Hz, then however powerful the aid and whatever its rated gain, the **s** will be almost—if not completely—inaudible. As a result, hearing impaired children capable of hearing this sound with appropriate amplification are simply never exposed to it. Now move the ruler to 5000 Hz, then 6000 Hz and see how much more information becomes available. The high frequency response of some wired systems can also be limited. This would be the case if the high frequency tone control is turned down perhaps to avoid whistling caused by acoustic feedback. If such whistling does occur, it is better to prevent it by reducing gain and increasing input than by reducing frequency range.

It was previously stated that each vowel has its own characteristic formant structure. While this is true, it does not follow that, on this account, the vowels will all sound different to hearing impaired children. By covering the frequencies above 1000 Hz in the spectrograms in Figure 14, we have seen that the second formants of the front vowels are obscured. Inspection of the remaining information shows that several of the vowels now look somewhat alike. For children with residual hearing extending only to 1000 Hz, these vowels also sound alike. Even to normal listeners, the vowel **ee** when low-pass filtered from 1000 Hz comes across as **oo**. In teaching speech or understanding why a hearing impaired child would make such confusions, it is essential to consider both the frequency range of the child's hearing and the frequency range of the aid. The fact that a sound is audible does not necessarily mean that it is discriminable. As the examples given show, most speech sounds are complex and the audibility of more than one component, e.g., vowel formant, is essential in speech sound identification.

Even within the frequency range available to hearing impaired children, auditory discrimination may not be as good as that of normal listeners. At low frequencies, hearing impaired listeners' discrimination of speech-like sounds may be normal, but as frequency increases, discrimination tends to become poorer than normal. However, frequency discrimination by hearing impaired children can be improved with training, and so can speech discrimination. What speech sounds any particular child can learn to discriminate must be determined pragmatically. For example, in a study by Doehring and the writer (19), children with little or no hearing over 1000 Hz who had failed to learn to discriminate between vowel sounds after several years in a strong auditory-oral program succeeded in learning such discrimination through programmed instruction. However, these children were not able to generalize from this training. When given the same words in a non-programmed test, they failed to identify the vowels previously learned. This finding shows the importance of making a distinction between discrimination and recognition of speech sounds, a point which will be discussed in a later section.

A phenomenon of great interest in relation to frequency range is the ability to identify many sounds which are inaudible in isolation but are identifiable in terms of the effect they have on adjacent phonemes. In Figure 14, one can see clearly that the consonants affect the vowels in predictable ways as the articulators move to or from the consonant via the vowel. To a hearing impaired child the vowel transitions, particularly if both F_1 and F_2 are audible, may be sufficient cues for the identification of, say, **p, t,** and **k.** The normally-hearing person certainly uses such vowel transition cues, but often in addition to other cues, such as the frequency of the burst when the consonant is released. To illustrate the point, say the words *cup* and *cut,* forming but not releasing the final consonant. Mask your face with a sheet or card to prevent identification of the sounds through lipreading. Then ask someone to tell you which word

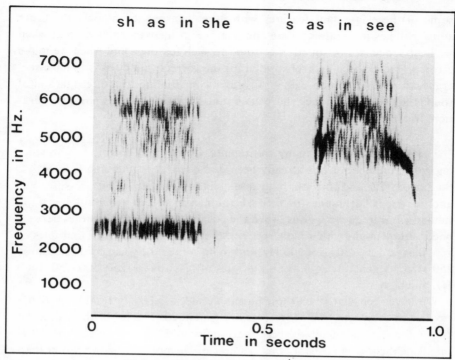

Figure   15. Spectrogram of s and sh.

was said. Recognition of the sounds, formed but not actually produced, is likely to be 100% correct because audible vowel transitions provide sufficient information to identify the adjacent, unreleased consonant. Some workers have found that such "hidden" auditory cues are better utilized by well trained and experienced hearing impaired persons than by normally-hearing listeners. Whether this is so or not, many such cues are available, and the ability of the hearing impaired person to use them serves to emphasize the need to teach speech sounds as part of a sequence rather than in isolation.

AUDITORY CUES AND FEATURE RECOGNITION

There is a notable lack of correspondence between phonemes as they are perceived and their acoustic patterns. For example, the acoustic characteristics of **k** preceding the vowel **ee** are quite different from those of **k** preceding the vowel **oo,** as we illustrated in Chapter I, Figure 9. To a person contrasting the whispered syllables **kee** and **koo** the differences are marked, the former being much higher in frequency than the latter. In spite of these differences, the two sounds, both heard as **k**, have many features in common and share some of these invariant features with other consonants, namely the other stops. Studies in aural encoding and short-term memory indicate that when we hear sequences of sounds we attend to such features, and when we make errors in recall the sound substituted for the correct sound tends to have several features in common with it. Features contributing to the recognition of sounds, some of which they share in common, include voicing, nasality, duration, frication, and place.

Voicing is common to many consonants. One of the acoustic cues to voicing, voice onset time, has already been discussed. A further cue is intensity, the unvoiced sounds having, in general, slightly greater sound pressure. Yet another cue is harmonic structure. Harmonics in speech are multiples of the fundamental frequency. Thus, when the vocal cords vibrate 125 times per second, as they might with a male speaker, they generate sounds at multiples of 125, that is, 125, 250, 375, 500 Hz, and so on. When the vocal cords vibrate at 250 Hz they generate sounds at multiples of 250, that is, 250, 500, 750, 1000 Hz, and higher.

We have seen that when these harmonics are selectively resonated by the cavities in the vocal tract, formants are generated. The lower the voice, the richer the speech sound will be in harmonics and the more clearly the formants defined. It is probably this richness of harmonic structure rather than the lower fundamental itself that leads to hearing impaired listeners commonly finding that the voiced sounds of low pitched speech are more intelligible than those of high pitched speech. The contrast between long duration voiced sounds which have harmonic structure and similar unvoiced sounds which are aperiodic generally causes little difficulty except for those with profound hearing impairment. For such listeners, the number of harmonics they are able to hear is limited, and for them, therefore, audibility of the fundamental appears to be important—not only because it can provide more information on intonation, but also because onset of a voiced consonant may also be cued by pitch changes.

In running speech, a further cue for discriminating between voiced and voiceless consonants is given by the breaks in the fundamental and higher harmonic structure. To the profoundly hearing impaired child these breaks may signal either an inaudible unvoiced consonant or a silent interval between words. On the basis of auditory information alone, the decision as to whether an inaudible consonant was present or not demands that other information—such as formant transitions, duration, rhythm, stress, and intonation—are taken into account. Reference to the breaks in the voicing bars shown in the spectrograms in Figure 14 indicates that, even for a listener with no hearing above 1000 Hz, such information is available. Its use by a hearing impaired child cannot, however, be learned unless he is trained to process sequences of sounds; for this cue, like many others, is not present in speech sounds heard in isolation.

Nasality is a feature common to **m, n,** and **ng.** The three major acoustic cues to nasality appear to be: (1) marked low frequency energy around 300 Hz of fairly long duration, (2) marked discontinuity of the formants in relation to adjacent sounds, and (3) the presence of ***antiformants,*** that is, regions of frequency where the harmonics of speech are suppressed, which occur immediately above the 300 Hz zone and in the area adjacent to F_2 of each nasal sound—about 1200 Hz for **m,** 1700 Hz for **n,** and 2000 Hz for **ng.** The strong low frequency energy and the discontinuities are clearly seen in the spectrograms presented in Figure 14. These cues have a common root in that when the nasal passages are coupled to the oral cavities by lowering the velum, the extra-large cavities and relatively small apertures result in abundant low frequency resonance, the oral cavities becoming free to resonate at their characteristic frequencies only when the velum is raised.

To learn to monitor the acoustic properties of the nasal sounds, therefore, the child requires adequate hearing for the low frequency components, ability to discern the characteristics of a pattern of sound versus silence over the frequency range in which the formants and antiformants occur, and ability to recognize the onset of vowel formants that are not continuant with the adjacent sound. Continuity and discontinuity effects can be clearly contrasted in Figure 14, where the low frequency semi-vowel **w** flows smoothly into the vowel $\overset{2}{\text{oo}}$ in the word *would,* but the vowel formants following **n** in *know,* and **m** in *more* and *must* appear suddenly at the termination of the nasal sound.

Hypernasality (nasal speech), as noted in Chapter VI, is often observed among hearing impaired children. This is generally related not to physical causes such as cleft palate, but to the child's inability to monitor his speech for nasalization through audition. In hypernasal speech the nasal sounds are usually poorly produced, but the acoustic structure of the vowels and other consonants is also weakened or distorted. Discontinuities between nasal sounds and nasalized vowels do not occur. Appropriate amplification—even for children who have hearing only for low frequencies—is, in the long run, an important means of preventing or treating hypernasality since the high energy sound at 300 Hz, the relative lack of energy immediately above this frequency, and the discontinuities between nasals and correctly produced adjacent back vowels are cues which are encompassed within their range of hearing. For children with a wider range of hearing the case for amplification is stronger since cues to nasality exist up to at least 2000 Hz. Adequate experience of listening to sound sequences is essential in developing auditory awareness of nasal/non-nasal distinctions. As with many other sounds, the cue which may be of greatest importance—in this case discontinuity—is simply not available to the child if sounds are taught in isolation.

The relative duration and onset characteristics of sounds also provide cues to their identity. Thus, nasal sounds are relatively long-duration consonants because their production requires the lowering and raising of the velum. This cannot be accomplished in the time required to form and release a stop-plosive. The sounds s and **t** have very similar frequency characteristics, but the s is much longer. If s is recorded on tape and the initial segment removed, then it is heard as a **t** on playback. The same is true for the sounds **w** and **b.** Duration is one of the primary cues distinguishing s, **z, sh,** and **zh** from the other, shorter fricative sounds. Duration cues may also determine whether sounds are heard as voiced or unvoiced. In the spectrograms shown in Figure 14, the "s" in *ease* is actually unvoiced, although heard as a **z.** This is because the preceding vowel, **ee,** is long in comparison with the s. If, for a further example, one whispers the words *peace* and *peas,* no actual voicing occurs, but each of the two words can be identified on the basis of the relative duration of the vowel and consonant. Relative duration can, of course, be judged only in sequences of sounds. Its use as a cue must depend on considerable experience in hearing sequences of speech, the patterns of which have a predictable rhythm.

Frication, a feature common to s, **z, sh,** and **f,** requires hearing in the frequency range above 2000 Hz for its detection. Hearing impaired children usually have considerably reduced sensitivity over this range of frequencies. Because the energy of fricative sounds is generally weaker than that of other sounds, they tend either to omit, distort, or substitute alternatives for these sounds. Problems associated with the audibility of certain fricatives caused by the restricted range of some hearing aids have already been discussed.

The *place* at which articulation occurs in the vocal tract is signaled by various acoustic cues. The most important of these are consonant-to-vowel or vowel-to-consonant transitions. While most of the other acoustic cues discussed above yield information on how a sound is produced, that is, whether the adjacent sound is a plosive or fricative, the direction of formant change provides cues as to which plosive or fricative has occurred. The way formant transitions help normal listeners to discriminate between **p, t,** and **k** has already been discussed, but other cues as to place of production contribute to the recognition of many consonants. Thus, the frequency of the noise burst associated with the release of the stops **p, t, k, b, d,** and **g** also helps us to identify them, and fricative sounds may be largely differentiated by their center frequencies as well as by their relative intensities. Similarly, nasal sounds are differentiated by the relative frequency of their second formants and antiformants as well as by the way they affect adjacent vowels.

Many cues on place of articulation are less audible to a hearing impaired child than cues on manner of articulation. Accordingly, more sounds which differ in place than differ in manner are confused by such children. The principle that one should work from the known to the unknown, the easy to the difficult, seems to be supported in relation to manner and place differences in speech teaching. If the manner of production is established first and then place features are superimposed on manner, one usually meets with more success than if following the reverse course. In other words, teaching the use of plosives in the order **b, d,** then **g** and the nasals **m, n,** then **ng** is usually more effective than teaching **b** then **m, d** then **n, g** then **ng,** etc.

ACOUSTIC CUES, HEARING AIDS, and HEARING LEVELS

We have seen that second formants of vowels are important to their identification and that second formant transitions can also provide important cues to the place of production of adjacent consonants. Since the F_2 of any vowel carries so much information, it is essential that it be rendered audible, if possible, to all hearing impaired children. The intensity of F_2 in relation to the remaining components of the vowel, to the response characteristics of a child's hearing aid, and to his hearing level is therefore of considerable importance. In the sentence depicted in the spectrograms of Figure 14, the peak sound pressure level of the vowels as measured two yards from the speaker fell within the range of 65 to 70 dB. The sound pressure level (SPL) of the first formant of these vowels was from 3 to 5 dB less than the peak levels. However, some of the F_2 levels were considerably less. Whereas F_2 for the vowel **a(r)** as in *art* was only 5 dB less than peak value of 70 dB, F_2 for **oo** as in *who* was 15 dB below the peak level of 65 dB, and F_2 of **ee** as in *ease* was 20 dB below the peak level of 68 dB. These differences between overall SPL of vowels and the SPL of their second formants are quite usual. They approximate the differences which would be found for most speakers. The back vowel **oo** would have an F_2 about 15 dB weaker than peak value, and as the vowels in the sentence approach the center vowels, the differences between F_2 and peak value would decrease gradually to about 5 dB and then increase again until, in the front vowel **ee,** the difference would be about 20 dB.

The above data in relation to formant intensities has been given in dB relative to .0002 dynes/square centimeter (SPL). But unlike the equipment used to measure sound pressure level, the ear does not have a flat response: it is more sensitive to sound in the mid frequency range than to sounds of either low or high frequency. Thus, the sound pressure level of low or high frequency sounds has to be greater than that for the mid frequency sounds in order to be audible to the normal listener. The point at which a pure tone of a given frequency becomes audible to normal listeners is represented on an audiogram as 0 dB hearing level (HL). The SPL equivalent to audiometric zero (0 dB HL) for each frequency (re ANSI, 1969, standard) is given at the bottom of the audiogram shown in Figure 16. By defining the center frequency of each formant and subtracting the difference between SPL and HL for that frequency for the measured intensity, one can convert the data on vowel components given above and show the approximate frequency and intensity location of each on an audiogram. This has been done for F_1 and F_2 of the vowels o͡o, a(r), and ee and for the consonants sh and s̓. The results are expressed in Figure 16 (IPA /u/, /a/, /i/, /ʃ/ and /s/). This figure shows that F_1 of the vowels o͡o and ee are very close in both intensity and frequency (about 40 dB HL at 250 to 270 Hz) and that the second formant of ee has slightly less intensity than the sound sh, but approximately the same center of frequency. The formants of the vowel a(r) are both louder than the other sounds and s̓ is the quietest and highest frequency sound of those presented.

Earlier it was stated that, because the normal ear was not equally sensitive to all frequencies, the first two vowel formants were heard at approximately the same *sensation level* (the level above the listener's threshold at which a signal is delivered). Reference to Figure 16 shows that this is so, the difference between F_1 and F_2 of any three vowels being no more than about 8 dB HL. But to the hearing impaired person this is not so. To a child with a hearing loss as depicted at the bottom of Figure 16, none of the sounds, unless it were amplified, would be audible. Even if the speaker halved the distance and thus increased the level of the sounds by 6 dB they would not be heard by a child with this audiogram. By adding 6 dB for every halving of distance it can be seen that sounds falling below 2000 Hz would become audible when the speaker's mouth was an inch or so from the ear. In this position the breath stream would also give tactile information to the hearing impaired child; speaking thus into the ear has been shown to be an effective means of providing auditory-tactile experience in the teaching of speech.

The response characteristics of a typical body-worn hearing aid which might be selected for a child with such an audiogram are shown in Figure 17. The curve shown was obtained with an input of 70 dB SPL (about the level of the vowels as spoken in Figure 14) and gain was near maximum. As with all hearing aid frequency response curves, the reference level was .0002 dynes/square centimeter. From this graph it is possible to determine (a) how much gain is provided at each frequency and (b) how much output is obtain-

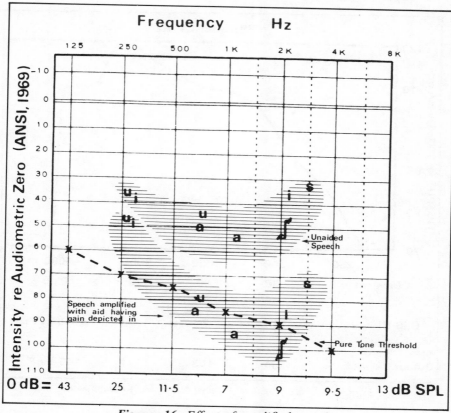

Figure 16. Effect of amplified speech.

able with a 70 dB input. The amount of gain can be read directly from the vertical axis: at 250 Hz, it is 10 dB, at 500 Hz, 30 dB and so on. The remaining figures are provided below the chart. To relate output to the audiogram, conversion to dB HL is required. To make this conversion the SPL equivalent to 0 dB HL is subtracted for each frequency. The results of these subtractions are also shown below the chart.

Now let us put together the data shown in Figures 16 and 17 so that we have a hypothetical hearing impaired child whose audiogram for the better ear is shown, a sample of speech, and a hearing aid to provide amplification. Which of the sounds thus spoken will the child hear with a hearing aid like this? The levels attained by adding the gain provided to the HL of the sounds are depicted as aided speech in Figure 16. It can be seen that only three elements of the utterance become audible: the two formants of **a(r)** and the **sh.** These are among the most powerful of the speech sounds, and it may be assumed that if these sounds are barely audible then the majority of other con-

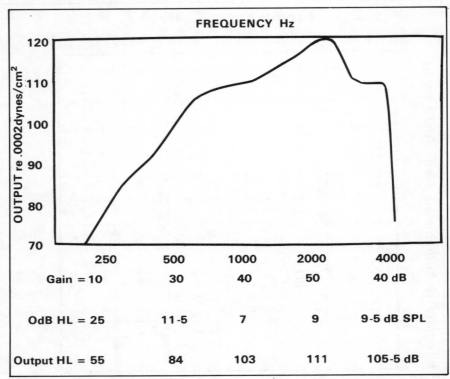

Figure 17. Response of typical body-worn hearing aid.

sonants and the acoustic cues which permit their identification will not be heard.

Technically, the hearing aid characteristics in Figure 17 show an average gain of 40 dB (the average gain at 500, 1000, and 2000 Hz), but this does not bring into our hypothetical child's auditory range the lower frequency sounds which occur within 30 dB of threshold. The center vowels are commonly observed in the vocalization and babble of hearing impaired children who have not received speech teaching, whereas the high back and high front vowels are not. It would seem likely that this more frequent use of center vowels is closely related to the type of amplification generally provided. We have seen that only two of the sounds as spoken, **a(r)** and **sh,** are audible to our child through this particular hearing aid. But what if the sounds were spoken closer to the microphone and input level were thus increased? Reduction of distance from 2 yards to 18 inches would result in a 12 dB increase. If 12 dB is added to the gain of the aid and each sound is then replotted, it can be seen that the majority of the sounds are still at threshold. Further decrease of distance or increase in speech level would probably cause output distortion. In other words, this hearing aid—if provided for a child with such an audiogram—is inappropriate. A more powerful model must be selected. The model selected must, clearly, provide better amplification for the low frequencies as well as for the high. In short, it must have a wider frequency range. Another hearing aid chosen simply in terms of a higher average gain over the frequencies 500, 1000, and 2000 Hz may prove equally inappropriate.

The above discussion indicates that an audiogram can help in the selection of a hearing aid; but, at best, audiograms show only the threshold of audibility. They tell more about what a child cannot hear than what he can. We listen to speech not at the threshold of audibility, but at levels well above threshold. It is the quality of hearing above threshold that largely determines how well we will perceive speech. But there is more to hearing than meets the ear. The skilled listener also appears actively to select information regarding variance and invariance of sound according to previous adaptive experience. The effects of listening experience are clearly demonstrated by comparing a child who is born with severe hearing impairment and one who loses hearing after acquiring speech and language. They may have identical audiograms but the performance of the latter is likely to be much superior. Thus the ability of a child to process sounds arriving above threshold cannot be predicted simply from an audiogram.

A further limitation relating to the use of an audiogram in hearing aid selection is that mid or high frequency thresholds which lie above 110 dB cannot be charted (or measured with most audiometers). Nevertheless, ability to hear at such intensities may be extremely important since, with appropriate amplification, sound well above 110 dB HL can be delivered to the ear. In cases where tolerance is no problem, such high levels of amplification may permit a child with little apparent hearing according to an audiogram to utilize some high frequency acoustic cues in the perception and production of speech. In contrast, the low frequency limits of most audiometers approach the threshold of tactile sensation, and response to low frequency sounds of high intensity which can be charted on an audiogram may represent tactile response rather than hearing.

There are, of course, children who are known to be hearing impaired for whom reliable audiograms cannot be obtained. This group includes infants. Since input levels are likely to vary considerably more than the approximate hearing levels, which can usually be established in such cases, there is no sound audiological reason to justify obtaining an accurate audiogram before selecting a hearing aid. With infants, we must either be prepared to select hearing aids on the basis of approximate information or lose valuable time.

Hearing Aid Selection and Auditory Training

The rationale underlying hearing aid selection has already been presented; and the need for amplification which provides adequate gain, frequency range, and output in relation to tolerance levels has been described. The procedure by which each child's hearing levels can be related to the amplification provided by a particular hearing aid has also been shown. But in selecting and using hearing aids there are many other points to take into account: body-worn versus head-worn personal aids, earmolds, monaural versus binaural fitting, the type and extent of training and experience a child requires in order to use amplification effectively—the list is not exhaustive.

For children whose hearing levels are stable and who require output levels up to 100-110 dB SPL, appropriate head-worn instruments may be recommended, since many hearing aids designed to be worn behind the ear or incorporated in glasses are equivalent or superior to body-worn instruments in terms of their acoustic characteristics. In general the less severely hearing impaired the child, the more suitable a head-worn aid is likely to be. This is because acoustic feedback is not likely to occur at output levels of 105 dB SPL or less even when the earmold fits poorly and the microphone of the aid is close to the receiver. For children who require output levels of less than 100 dB—particularly those with sloping audiograms—head-worn aids with vented ear molds can be used, since below 100 dB SPL feedback is no longer a problem. With open or vented molds, high frequency sounds arrive at the eardrum via the mold, while the low frequency sounds arrive unamplified, via the opening in the mold. The two sources add together to make a fairly complete and intelligible pattern. Open or vented molds appear to be superior to closed molds for listening to speech in noise. If the child can be relied upon to care for his hearing aid and meets the requirements outlined above, then head-worn rather than body-worn aids should be selected.

Body-worn aids with closely fitting molds are essential to the more severely hearing impaired child because such children require high output levels and good low frequency response: Earmolds for severely hearing impaired children wearing body-type aids should preferably have a long meatal projection in order to ensure a good seal. Children usually manage best when the molds are made of soft, pliable material because they allow more comfort when chewing and are less likely to cause cuts or bruises if—as often happens—the child falls on, or otherwise receives a blow to, his ear. In a survey undertaken some years ago, the writer found that children with soft molds made considerably more consistent and effective use of their hearing aids than did children with hard molds because these hazards were avoided. To prevent noise due to clothes rub and physical damage to the instrument, body-worn hearing aids should be securely harnessed. Priority in selection should be given to those hearing aids that can best withstand the physical beating to which children often expose them. Water, sand, soup, food, hard blows to the casing, and resulting jolts to the circuitry are daily perils to which hearing aids are subjected, particularly by the young. Few aids can stand such assault and continue to function.

Two hearing aids should in theory yield better results than one. The use of two ear-level hearing aids which can move with the head are thought to facilitate localization, and ability to localize sound through the use of head-worn hearing aids has been demonstrated with adults. An acoustic shadow, amounting to about 13 dB for some frequencies, occurs when the head intervenes between a single ear-level aid and the source of a sound. The use of two head-worn hearing aids clearly prevents the attenuation of sound through head shadow. An effect known as interaural summation occurs when two ears are stimulated rather than one. This results in an increase in sensitivity in the order of 3-6 dB. Body-worn hearing aids, one to each ear, may not permit localization and are subject to body baffle effects, but they do contribute to total input through interaural summation.

Whether two hearing aids are better than one for a particular child has to be determined pragmatically. One tries both conditions and makes judgments on the basis of the child's responses to speech in the course of training. In some cases, even when differences in pure tone hearing level between ears are minimal, binaural as compared to monaural hearing aids have been shown to *detract* from the intelligibility of speech. While significant differences among binaural, pseudo-binaural (Y-cord), and monaural hearing aids for children have not been demonstrated through well controlled studies, most clinical and educational experience suggests that two aids are superior to one. In the absence of acceptable experimental data either way, clinicians and teachers who fit binaurally justify this on the grounds that binaural fitting is unlikely to affect the child adversely while monaural fitting might be detrimental if the aid is fitted to what might turn out to be the poorer ear for speech perception. An adequate comparison of binaural and monaural conditions requires that the best possible selection of aids has been made for the individual children studied. But neither the procedures used in selecting aids nor the tests that are used in making such comparisons have been sufficiently developed. Until reliable and valid procedures and tests are available, the relative merits of binaural and monaural fitting for any child must remain in question.

Auditory training for speech perception and production is a subject which requires considerable attention. There are many drill books and suggestions for teachers available (7, 12, 31, 49, 64, 78, 89), but so little experimental work has been done that the possibilities and limitations of auditory training are not fully known. Looking back over previous sections of this chapter, it can be seen that a number of skills must be developed if the patterns of speech are to be understood or monitored efficiently in quiet (let alone noisy) conditions. These would include: discrimination between presence or absence of sound and between loud-quiet, high-low, long-short, sudden-gradual, simple-complex, steady-changing, etc.; ability to use information given by rhythm, stress, intonation, number and rate of syllables, etc.; capacity to code, retain, and recall the sequential order of phonemes, words, and sentences spoken; and ability to supply information relative to inaudible items in a sequence on the basis of a knowledge of language acquired through previous adaptive experience. It would appear that auditory programs should at least provide training in these specific skills.

A large number of programs studied by the writer include training in some of these skills. Many also follow the principle of proceeding from gross to fine differences, and in some programs it is assumed that there is a certain hierarchy in the skills involved. Many programs of training begin with discrimination between grossly different non-speech sounds: bells, drums, whistles, horns, etc. While this can be highly entertaining and may encourage the child to listen, does it really help in the processing of speech sounds? Non-speech sounds tend to be of much longer duration than speech and have different onset characteristics and frequency distribution. They may be more grossly different than some speech sounds, but they may also be so different from speech that there is no carry-over. This would, in the light of research on dichotic listening, seem to be the case. Speech tends to be processed in one hemisphere of the brain and non-speech sounds in the other.

Experiments indicate that recall of verbal and nonverbal sequences by hearing impaired children involves different perceptual and memory processes. It would therefore seem logical, if one is attempting to develop better auditory perception and monitoring of speech, to work from gross to fine differences within the speech mode. It would not appear difficult to rank order acoustic features which characterize the vowels and consonants according to extent of difference on several parameters, but in doing so it is important to bear in mind what features are likely to be audible to the particular child being trained. As with speech teaching, auditory training should involve a considerable amount of work geared to the individual.

There are several dangers in considering discrimination among items in a small set (for example, among two or three words differing by specific features or phonemes) to be evidence that the child can utilize the cues that distinguish them from others. Under conditions where the set is limited, a child may quickly learn to discriminate among items, but the cues which the child uses in order to make the discrimination may be irrelevant to the absolute identification of the sound in question. For example, a child may produce a lateralized $\overset{\mathsf{I}}{\mathsf{s}}$ which sounds rather like **sh**. The teacher may decide to have the child listen to two patterns, **sha(r)** and **sa(r)** presented randomly, and require the child to show her which of the sounds she makes by pointing to a card on which the two syllables are written. The technique is in common use. Now assume that the frequency range of the child's hearing aid allows him to hear the **sh** but not the $\overset{\mathsf{I}}{\mathsf{s}}$. The child could score 100% correct on such discriminations simply on the basis that the **sh** was audible but the $\overset{\mathsf{I}}{\mathsf{s}}$ was not. This training could even help him produce the sound in the teaching situation, but it would not have taught him to identify the $\overset{\mathsf{I}}{\mathsf{s}}$ or to monitor his production of it through hearing.

A similar danger in teaching children auditory discrimination within small sets is that the child may identify the sounds by a process of elimination. If three words differing only in the final phoneme are presented, such as *dog, doll,* and *dot,* the child who knows only *dog* and *doll* can succeed in identifying *dot* with 100% accuracy by adopting the strategy of pointing to the one which is not known (or in which the final sound is not audible). This type of training clearly does not lead to absolute identification of the **t**. Even when the required sounds are presented in different sets so that the teacher is sure that discriminations are being made on the basis of meaningful cues, discriminations are still relative to the size of the sets used in the training.

An analogy might be drawn from common experience. Most people have at some time met a person in the street whose face is sufficiently familiar to justify a nod, smile, or other greeting, but about whom no identifying information can be recalled. Subsequent experience might tell us that the person was the bank clerk. That he was recognized in one context but not in another would be analogous to discrimination within a set. In contrast, recognizing the bank clerk at a chance meeting in Hong Kong or Timbuktu, a feat of memory requiring thorough familiarity with the clerk's distinguishing features, could be considered an example of absolute identification.

Some hearing impaired children do no more than discriminate between some of the sounds of speech on the basis of missing cues or by the process of elimination, but this would not be true for all hearing impaired children or for all sounds. There are usually a number of sounds which can be absolutely identified, perceived categorically, by all but the most profoundly deaf children. The basic requirement for their absolute identification or certain production is overlearning, which might be described as the stage in training not when the child can get the item right but when he cannot get it wrong. The required level of sophistication is probably attainable only if extensive experience complements training (and vice-versa). Full use of amplification for speech under the best possible conditions in and out of school is essential in providing adequate experience.

A case has been made for unisensory training in which the hearing impaired child is required to discriminate or identify speech samples without lipreading. The case for unisensory training is based on the rationale that simultaneous attention to the information provided in two channels will detract from the amount of information yielded by either. The writer knows of no satisfactory experimental evidence in support of the notion, *but* on the basis of his own and others' experience in teaching hearing impaired children, he favors a unisensory (auditory) approach as a means of developing residual hearing. Such auditory training, provided regularly as part of a well structured program, appears to prepare certain children to be more flexible in the strategies they adopt in communicating with others in real life situations. Initial unisensory auditory training seems, in other words, to permit better use of the two main sources of live information—hearing and lipreading—under conditions which demand the use of both.

Checks of Hearing Aid Function

Daily checks on hearing aids are the only way to ensure that they function properly. The simplest form of check is to listen to an aid oneself and to ensure that the whole gamut of speech sounds is reproduced clearly. To check personal aids, one needs a custom fitted earmold, since low frequencies are lost unless the receiver is coupled perfectly to the ear. For the purpose of such a check, the hearing aid should be adjusted to provide as much output as one can tolerate comfortably, since this approaches the power output required by the child.

As the previous discussion indicates, testing with the sentence and sounds shown in Figure 14, spoken with constant vocal effort, will permit the teacher to determine whether reproduction over the required frequency range is adequate. Each vowel should sound about as loud as any other, although slightly louder central vowels are normal since the vocal tract is less restricted in their production. Any aid which reproduces certain vowels which peak in energy much above the others or are distorted should be rejected and serviced. In addition to the sentence, the sounds **sh** and **s̬** should be employed to check that the aid functions well over the high frequency (2000 to 4000 Hz) range. All hearing aids should reproduce both sounds. In Figure 15, these sounds spoken in isolation were deliberately produced at a greater intensity than they would have been in running speech. The **sh** and **s̬** used to test the aid should not be louder than those which occur in running speech. If the **s̬** of the type you normally produce in running speech is quiet to you or inaudible through the aid, then it will certainly not be heard, or reproduced spontaneously, by the child.

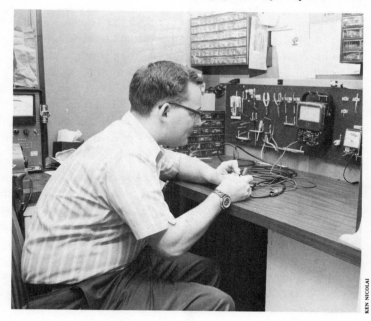

Checking a hearing aid.

As mentioned earlier, it is unlikely that the s̍ will sound entirely natural through a personal aid, but it is essential that enough of its components are reproduced for the sound to be identified without difficulty.

The listener making this check should be able to detect whether the instrument generates an undesirable level of hum (often found in wired systems), hiss (usually associated with poor quality transistors), or distortion of one sort or another. Distortion can occur in each stage of a hearing aid system (input, amplifier, or output) and in the coupling of components. For example: microphones may be accidentally dropped or treated roughly and, as a result, work poorly; a smoothing condenser in the main amplifier of a wired system may cause hum; receivers or earphones may become damaged; or wires may fracture with use and cause crackle or intermittent reception. In loop induction or radio systems the loop patterns or antennae position may result in patchy transmission or "dead" spots where reception simply cannot occur. Thus it is important for the teacher of speech not only to check the aid, but to check it under the conditions in which she teaches. Elementary errors, such as teaching through loop induction when the child is seated directly in the dead spot located under a suspended loop, are thus avoided. Such "on the spot" checks can also indicate to the teacher the effects of clothes rub (which results when the microphone of the system is too loosely harnessed), dragging the wire of a microphone over obstacles while talking to the child, allowing direct breath stream to strike the microphone, overloading, etc.

Perhaps the most important check that a teacher can make on a hearing aid's function is through close observation of the child's responses to auditory stimuli. While checking the aid is essential, so too is thinking of the aid as an integral part of the child's auditory system. One should seek to establish not only a consistency of hearing aid usage, but a consistency of response to sound, so that changes in response may signal breakdown somewhere in the system which begins at the microphone of the aid and ends at the cortex. For example, sudden changes in middle ear pressure, perhaps due to an allergy or cold, may be reflected by reduced responsivity to sound.

Battery failure provides an example of analogous breakdown in the hearing aid part of the auditory system. Most batteries used in modern hearing aids are cells of the silver oxide or mercury type. Silver oxide batteries provide higher voltage and greater milliwatt-hour ratings (longer life) than other existing batteries of the same size. They start their life providing a certain voltage, usually 1.6v, and maintain about 1.5v until the cell is exhausted. At this point, the voltage drops suddenly. It is possible to begin a speech lesson with adequate battery power yet have a silver oxide cell die before the lesson is completed. In contrast, mercury batteries rated as 1.3v start their life at this level, drop by about 0.1v over the first quarter of their life, and then maintain a constant voltage until they are almost exhausted. They decline fairly gradually over their last five hours of life. Most aids begin to distort as batteries drop in power. The expected life of a cell is calculated in relation to the current each hearing aid requires, and such data are usually provided in the manufacturer's specifications.

Teachers and parents alert to such matters will save themselves considerable frustration and do much to ensure the consistency of auditory input the child requires by making adequate arrangements for battery replacement. Similar changes in response may occur if earmolds become blocked with wax. Such checks as those described above may be regarded as subjective, but their validity is beyond question since the hearing aid is only one aspect of the complete system in which all parts must work effectively.

More objective tests on hearing aids should also be routinely undertaken by technicians using appropriate instruments to measure and record how the hearing aid functions. Such equipment should be available in a nearby center if not directly in the school. Experience suggests that one skilled technician should be available for every 100 hearing impaired children to check and maintain their hearing aids in adequate condition. But, however much technical help is available, the responsibility for ensuring that the hearing aid is appropriate to the child and in good working condition rests squarely upon the person responsible for teaching speech to the child.

CHAPTER IV

Instructional Analysis of Consonants and Vowels

In this chapter we proceed from Dr. Ling's treatment of the use of the auditory system through amplification to all the sensory possibilities for production of the sounds of speech. Anticipating the discussion of methods in Chapters V and VI, we present information and suggestions about phonemes and combinations of phonemes that have direct application to the instructional process. Our treatment of phonemes on an individual basis does not imply a way of teaching. Rather it is to equip the teacher with an understanding of units basic to the production of speech and their dynamics as they are influenced by coarticulation, described in Chapter I. For example, we are aware that the **p** that initiates a syllable is different from the **p** in the word *speech*. In the initiating case there is a discernible explosion, and in the other case the production is shorter and almost voiced—not quite exploded. Contrast the production of **p** in the words *peach* and *speech*; similarly, *tore* and *store, cool* and *school*.

For certain phonemes—particularly vowels—there may be variations in production, that is, the vowel boundaries related to sectionalisms may be quite extensive. Here our recommendation is to make the best approximation to general American production, and to accept that which is intelligible and which is easily produced by the child. For example, for the word *cent* some people may say **cint** and some may call it **cent**. Here we leave it to the teacher's judgment as to which can best be produced by the child. Another illustration is the diphthongization of vowels by Southern talkers. The general American talker pronounces the word *bed* as **bed** while the Southern talker may diphthongize it as **beud**.

What we have selected about phonemes for inclusion in this chapter, although not exhaustive, constitutes a broad and solid foundation to devise and apply techniques appropriate to a child's requirements, whether for development or correction of individual sounds or their combinations. For each phoneme there are symbols of the Northampton system, of the International Phonetic Alphabet, and of Webster's dictionary. Key words are presented along with some unusual spellings to remind the teacher about transformations to the primary spelling. We then describe the production of each phoneme, including conventional shorthand descriptions used in the phonetic literature.

This is followed by the internal sensory feedback readily available to the speaker, that is, what is available to the feedback system the child carries around with him. An example is the motor feedback he gets whenever he speaks, unlike the feedback he may get from a mirror which is not an integral part of him. Given our aim to have the child speak in real-life situations, which requires monitoring his own production, we emphasize the importance of internal feedback.

We then analyze instructional possibilities for communicating the properties of the phoneme visually, tactually, and, wherever possible, auditorily. Suggestions and alternative techniques for development grow out of these analyses. We then list the probable errors of deaf talkers and suggestions for remediation. The probabilities include *large class errors* such as voice and voiceless confusion, *subclass errors* such as those that may have to do with excessive pressure occurring in plosives, and errors that may be *singular for a particular phoneme* such as the place variations determined by phonetic context in the production of **k**.

Consonants are ordered following the vertical columns of the Northampton Consonant Chart (Figure 2) and follow the order in Table 1. The vowels are presented in the order in Table 2 and are grouped as back round, front, mid back, mixed, and diphthongs.

h-

h- /h/ h-

KEY WORDS: **h**ad, a**h**ead
SPELLINGS: h, **wh**(o)

Production *(oral breath/voiced fricative)*

Nasopharyngeal port closes, breath is directed through the oral cavity—which assumes the configuration for the following vowel—with audible friction. The **h-** has no oral cavity formation of its own but changes with the vowels which surround it (**h-** is always followed by a vowel). In an intervocalic position (*ahead*), **h-** is commonly produced as a voiced fricative. The production of audible friction, while the oral cavity assumes the position for surrounding vowels, distinguishes the **h-** sound. Audible friction may be caused somewhat at the glottis by turbulence around the vocal folds, but to a large extent by breath rushing through the oral cavity across the tongue, velum, and palate. The relative lack of constriction in most vowel formations requires that breath be emitted with greater force than for other fricatives in order to make it audible.

Internal Feedback Information

TACTILE: Some friction from restricted breath flow on the tongue, velum, and palate.

KINESTHETIC: Some thoracic muscular tensing in emitting breath with sufficient force for audibility.

Sensory Instructional Possibilities

TACTILE: Steady breath flow on skin of the hand.

VISUAL: Steady breath flow by movement of feather, flame, paper.

Suggestions for Development

1. Develop in syllables using different vowels following **h-**. Have the student produce a series of **hee hee hee hee hee** on a single breath so that the **h-** is audible, but without running out of breath. Then have him produce a series of **h-**sounds with other vowels. When each vowel can be made in combination with

h- in a series without running out of breath, have the student produce a series on a single breath, mixing vowel sounds as follows: **hee hoo haw ha(r) hu-**. Demonstrate by lines drawn under the written symbols that the **h-** is relatively short in duration compared to the vowel sound.

2. Have the student feel the flow of breath on his hand. Associate with the written "h." Use a feather, strip of paper, or other visual aid only if necessary to demonstrate flow of breath. *Avoid* giving the impression of a sudden puff of breath, dropping the jaw, or exaggerating the force of production.

3. Develop in intervocalic positions as a voiced fricative. In such phrases as, "I have —," demonstrate that the voicing continues by drawing a continuous line under the phrase and let the student feel with his hand that the teacher's voice does not stop. Demonstrate the increased force of air emitted at the **h-** position by letting the child feel the emission with his other hand. The voice **h-** may be written "ħ" to remind the student of voicing.

4. Demonstrate the nature of the voiced friction by associating the **ħ** with other voiced fricatives; practice a series **v ħ ħ**, feeling the emission of slight breath on each.

Common Errors and Suggestions for Improvement

1. Excessive breath emitted: Use cool mirror close to student's mouth to show excess breath on **h-** (by breath moisture condensation). Compare with teacher's acceptable production. Produce a series of syllables with **h** followed by a vowel (**hee hee hee**) for student to practice controlling breath emission. Increase the number of syllables with practice. For the intervocalic **h-**, practice a continuously voiced string of syllables (**heeheeheehee**). Demonstrate graphically the need for a reduced **h-** production by writing the "h" smaller than the vowel or by underlining the "h" and the vowel so that the "h" line is shorter.

2. Insertion of -u- between h- and the following vowel: Have student practice taking position for the following vowel before producing **h-**. Demonstrate graphically by substituting a dotted line symbol for the vowel in place of the "h" symbol, as in the word *ham* written as "ːam."

3. Excessive friction with lingua-velar restriction: To gain tactile feedback the student may elevate the back of the tongue to approximate the velum for **h-**, giving a harsh or guttural sound (like clearing the throat). Redevelop with the vowel **ee** for which the front of the tongue is elevated. Let the student feel the inappropriate vibrations under the chin near the base of the tongue; contrast with **h-** produced with no vibrations.

wh

wh   /ʍ/   hw

KEY WORDS: **wh**en, every**wh**ere
SPELLINGS: wh, (t)w-, (s)w-

Production *(bilabial breath fricative)*

No voice, nasopharyngeal port closes, the lips are rounded as in the vowel oo and slightly protruded. Breath is directed through the oral cavity and the constricted opening of the lips with audible friction. Lip protrusion and roundings are less tense than for the vowel oo or for **w-**. Rounding and protruding the lips tends to raise the back of the tongue.

Internal Feedback Information

TACTILE: Friction of restricted breath flow on the rounded lips.

KINESTHETIC: Rounding and protruding of lips.

Sensory Instructional Possibilities

TACTILE: Steady breath flow on skin of the hand.

VISUAL: Rounding and protruding of lips. Steady breath flow by movement of feather, flame, strip of paper.

Suggestions for Development

1. Imitate from teacher's model; *avoid* giving the impression of a sudden puff of breath.

2. Demonstrate the flow of breath by tactile impression on student's hand.

3. Demonstrate the flow of breath by visual impression with *steady* deflection of a strip of paper, feather, or candle flame.

4. With student and teacher seated side-by-side, show in a mirror the degree of rounding and protrusion of lips. *Avoid* giving the impression of tense lip rounding and protrusion.

5. To demonstrate steady but not excessive flow of breath, have the young student attempt to blow out a series of seven or eight candles on a single breath. *Avoid* having the student take a deep breath to accomplish this.

Common Errors and Suggestions for Improvement

1. Excess force of expelled breath: Have student feel the contrasted breath flow for acceptable and unacceptable production on his hand. Use a mirror to demonstrate that the cheeks are not puffed out. Develop in syllables showing with underlining that the **wh** is shorter than the following vowel. Have student produce a series of syllables, such as **whee whee whee whee whee whee**, on a single breath for breath control.

2. Excess tension of the lips: Redevelop using a narrow but not rounded lip opening for **wh** production.

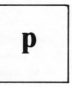

p /p/ p

KEY WORDS: **p**ie, si**p**, sto**pp**ed
SPELLINGS: p, pp

Production *(bilabial, breath stop)*

IMPLOSION: No voice, nasopharyngeal port closes, lips close, air is held and compressed in the oral cavity.

EXPLOSION: Air compressed in the oral cavity is exploded as audible breath between the lips. In connected speech, **p** is imploded and exploded in the initial position of words and syllables (*pie, helper*), and following **m** (*limp, ramp*) and ś (*lisp, rasp*) in the final position of words. It is imploded but not exploded preceding ś (*lips, caps*) or another stop consonant (*apt, crept*) in the same syllable, and following ś in the same syllable (*space, spot*). It is either not exploded or very lightly exploded in the final position (*sip, help*).

Internal Feedback Information

TACTILE: Lips touch with closure, exploded air between lips.

KINESTHETIC: Lips close with sufficient force to retain compressed air briefly.

Sensory Instructional Possibilities

TACTILE: Exploded air on skin of back of hand.

VISUAL: Lip closure and opening can be seen easily, explosion of air by movement of feather, flame, paper.

Suggestions for Development

1. Imitate from teacher's model; *avoid* dropping jaw with production.

2. Demonstrate manner of production by analogy from other plosives (note: **p** is frequently the first plosive developed).

3. Demonstrate explosion by tactile impression of breath on student's hand.

4. Demonstrate explosion by visual impression of sudden movement of strip of paper, feather, or candle flame; *avoid* exaggeration of force of explosion.

5. If necessary, manipulate for production by pushing on student's filled cheeks, press his lips together and open them rapidly, or stop his stream of blowing by occluding his lips and releasing.

6. Develop the imploded **p** after the imploded-exploded production is accomplished. Imitate from teacher's model of vowel interrupted by lip closure, as in **a(r)p**, without release of the compressed air.

7. Demonstrate the lack of movement of a strip of paper, feather, or candle flame on the imploded **p**; compare with exploded **p** with same visual aids.

8. Demonstrate by tactile analogy the difference between exploded **p** and imploded **p** by having the student press his palms together and release them quickly (exploded) or release them very gently (imploded).

9. Written symbols may indicate whether the **p** is exploded or imploded as follows: exploded "p-", imploded "p"; imploded **p** may be written in brackets as in "li[p]," may be outlined in dots, or may be written faintly; a short vertical "stop" line may be used for the non-exploded **p** as in "erup$_1$t" or "sip$_1$".

Common Errors and Suggestions for Improvement

1. Excess pressure on explosion of breath: If cheeks are puffed, show child appropriate production by mirror. Demonstrate reduced pressure by tactile impression of breath on student's hand. Contrast excess breath with appropriate amount. Have the student produce a series of rapid **p** sounds (**pppppppppp**) on the same breath; then a series of **pu- pu- pu- pu- pu-** syllables on a single breath.

2. Insufficient pressure on explosion of breath: Demonstrate increased pressure by tactile impression of breath on student's hand; use strip of paper or other visual aid. Contrast increased breath with insufficient amount. Demonstrate degree of pressure by pressing together student's thumb and forefinger or by pressing his hands together. Manipulate by lightly compressing child's lips together.

3. Escape of breath through nose on explosion: Demonstrate oral emission of breath by placing feather or strip of paper where it can be moved by oral but not nasal breath. Place card just under nose to separate oral and nasal breath emission; place bits of paper on top of card which will be moved by unwanted nasal breath. Place cool mirror under nose to show fogging with nasal breath. Having student close off both his nostrils with his thumb and forefinger while producing **p**, then produce **p** with nostrils open.

4. Dropping jaw on release of explosion: Use a mirror for imitation of teacher's correct production of **p** in isolation. Demonstrate student's faulty production by exaggeration; compare with appropriate production. Have the student produce series of syllables (**pee pee pee**), observing his productions in a mirror. There should be no dropping of the jaw. If necessary, the teacher may hold her hand under the student's jaw during production of **p** to prevent dropping of the jaw.

5. Substitution of **b** *for* **p,** *a sonant for surd error:* Write "b" and cross it out to make student aware of the nature of his error. Demonstrate the tactile difference by having student feel explosion of breath on **p** and voice vibration on **b.** Write a faint (or dotted) "h" in the space after "p" as in "pḥie." To extend duration of exploded **p,** demonstrate by writing the "p" with a line extended from it in a syllable, thus: "p___aw."

6. Blowing rather than imploded/exploded production: Demonstrate tactile difference on back of student's hand; demonstrate visual difference with feather or strip of paper.

$$\boxed{\textbf{t}}$$

t   /t/   t

KEY WORDS: tie, sit, sitting
SPELLINGS: t, tt, -ed,
Th-(Thomas)

Production *(lingua-alveolar breath stop)*

IMPLOSION: No voice, nasopharyngeal port closes, point of the tongue closes against alveolar ridge and side of tongue against molars, air is held and compressed in the oral cavity.

EXPLOSION: Air compressed in the oral cavity is exploded as audible breath between alveolar ridge and point of the tongue through slightly open teeth and lips.

In connected speech, t is imploded but not exploded preceding s̍ (*eats, bits*) and following s̍ in the same syllable (*stop, star*). It is both imploded and exploded in the initial position of syllables when followed by a vowel (*tie, retain*), following other lingua-alveolar consonants (*want, salt*), and other breath consonants (*kept, act, fast, watched*) in the final position of words. It is either not exploded or very lightly exploded in the final position of words (*bracelet, sit*).

Internal Feedback Information

TACTILE: Point of the tongue touches the alveolar ridge, exploded air is felt between tongue and alveolar ridge.

KINESTHETIC: Movement of tongue slightly upward to alveolar ridge.

Sensory Instructional Possibilities

TACTILE: Exploded air on skin of the hand.

VISUAL: Raised tongue point through the slightly open teeth, explosion of air by movement of feather, flame, paper.

Suggestions for Development

1. Imitate from teacher's model; *avoid* dropping jaw with production.

2. Demonstrate manner of production by analogy from **p**.

3. Demonstrate explosion by tactile impression of breath on student's hand.

4. Demonstrate explosion by visual impression of sudden movement of strip of paper, feather, or candle flame; *avoid* exaggeration of force of articulation.

5. Demonstrate place of production by slowly giving a visual exaggeration of the formation: with teacher's mouth wide open, place tongue point behind upper teeth, slowly narrow opening (keeping tongue in place) toward normal position, and produce exploded **t**. Have student attempt to imitate this production with a mirror if he cannot produce it without.

6. Demonstrate manner and place of production by giving a visually exaggerated step-by-step production: form **t** with the tongue point outside the oral cavity making closure with front of the upper lip and explode; next make the closure with the tongue point on the lower edge of upper lip and explode; next make the closure on the upper teeth and finally on the alveolar ridge. Have the student imitate each step as the tongue is drawn back into the oral cavity.

7. Develop the imploded **t** after the imploded-exploded production is accomplished. Demonstrate with techniques that are similar to those suggested for the sound **p.**

Common Errors and Suggestions for Improvement

1. Excess pressure on explosion of breath: Demonstrate reduced pressure by tactile impression of breath on student's hand; contrast excess breath with appropriate amount. Demonstrate reduced pressure by tactile impression of teacher's thumb pressed against student's palm; contrast excess pressure with appropriate amount. Have the student produce a series of rapid **t** sounds (**tttttttttt**) on a single breath; then a series of **ta(r)** syllables, (**ta(r) ta(r) ta(r)**), or **tip** syllables, (**tip, tip, tip, tip, tip**) on a single breath.

2. Insufficient pressure on explosion of breath: Demonstrate increased pressure by tactile impression of breath on student's hand; use strip of paper, feather, or other visual aid. Demonstrate pressure by pressing together student's thumb and forefinger, or his hands, and releasing them.

3. Improper place of production (tip of tongue on back of upper teeth or mid-portion of tongue against alveolar ridge): Redevelop **t** using open mouth position to give visual information about position of point of tongue against alveolar ridge. Use diagram or model to show correct placement; have student use mirror to produce **t** with appropriate placement.

4. Dropping jaw on release of explosion: Have student produce series of syllables **tee tee tee tee**, observing his productions in a mirror. There should be no dropping of the jaw. Demonstrate with teacher's production of **ta(r) ta(r) ta(r)**, pointing out that the jaw does not drop. If jaw dropping persists, teacher may hold her hand under student's jaw as he produces syllables. Have student hold his own hand under his jaw for tactile feedback.

5. Substitution of **d** *for* **t,** *a sonant for surd error:* Write "d" and cross it out to make student aware of the nature of his error. Demonstrate the tactile difference by having student feel explosion of breath on **t** and voice vibration on **d**. To extend duration of exploded **t**, demonstrate by writing the "t" with a line extended from it in a syllable, thus: "t____oo."

6. Too wide a mouth opening on production: Have the student produce the series of syllables **tee tee tee** and **eet eet eet**, observing his productions in a mirror; there should be no movement of the jaw. The student may hold a pencil eraser between his teeth while producing these syllables to assure that the jaw does not drop. Practice production of **t** in association with **p** in syllables **ipitip, ipitip, ipitip.**

k /k/ k

KEY WORDS: **k**ey, ba**ck**, be**c**ome
SPELLINGS: k, c, -ck, cc,
ch(school), -(a)lk

Production *(lingua-velar breath stop)*

IMPLOSION: No voice, nasopharyngeal port closes, back of tongue closes against front portion of velum or back portion of palate, air is held and compressed in the back of the oral cavity. *Note:* the point of contact on the velum-palate changes with surrounding vowels.

EXPLOSION: Air compressed in the back of the oral cavity is exploded as audible breath between the velum-palate and back of the tongue through slightly open teeth and lips.

In connected speech, **k** is imploded but not exploded preceding $\overset{\shortmid}{s}$ (*cooks, talks*) or another stop consonant in the same syllable (*act, elect*), and following $\overset{\shortmid}{s}$ in the same syllable (*skin, scat*). It is both imploded and exploded in the initial position of words and syllables (*king, crow, declare*), and immediately following any consonant in the final position (*ask, bank, bark, milk*). It is either not exploded or very lightly exploded in the final position following a vowel (*like, sack*).

Internal Feedback Information

TACTILE: Closure of back of tongue on velum or palate gives little information.

KINESTHETIC: Raising of back of tongue to close against velum or palate gives little information.

Sensory Instructional Possibilities

TACTILE: Exploded air on skin of the hand.

VISUAL: Exploded air by movement of feather, flame, or paper; place of production visible only with exaggerated mouth opening.

Suggestions for Development

1. Imitate from teacher's model; *avoid* dropping jaw with production. *Note:*

fair to very poor sensory features make **k** a difficult sound to develop from imitation.

2. Demonstrate manner of production by analogy from **p** to **t**.

3. Demonstrate explosion by tactile impression of breath on student's hand.

4. Demonstrate explosion by visual impression of sudden movement of strip of paper, feather, or candle flame; *avoid* exaggeration of force of articulation.

5. Demonstrate place of production by slowly giving a visual exaggeration of the formation: with the teacher's mouth wide open, place the back of the tongue against the back portion of the palate (keeping the point of the tongue behind the lower front teeth), slowly narrow mouth opening (keeping tongue in place) toward normal position and explode **k**. Have student attempt to imitate this production, using a mirror if necessary.

6. Demonstrate manner and place of production by giving a visually exaggerated step-by-step production: form **k** with the back of the tongue against the back of the upper front teeth (keeping the point of the tongue behind the lower front teeth and explode (sound will be similar to **t**); next make the closure with the back of the tongue on the alveolar ridge and explode; next closure on the front portion of the palate and finally on the back portion of the palate. Have the student imitate each step as the back of the tongue is drawn back into the oral cavity.

7. Develop **k** in association with the **ee** vowel, a position in which the tongue is very close to the velum-palate, helping to avoid dropping the jaw on production of **k**. Closure of the **k** on syllables **eek** or **kee** is likely to be at the back of the palate rather than on the velum, avoiding unwanted noise of closure on the back of the velum and uvula.

8. While the student attempts to produce **t**, hold the tip of his tongue down (with finger or tongue blade) behind the lower front teeth (do not let the back of the tongue move forward). Associate the exploded sound he produces with written "k." After several repetitions with the teacher or student holding down the tip of the tongue, have the student attempt the production without this aid.

9. Have the seated student hold his mouth slightly open and breathe deeply through his nose (to accomplish this the velum and back of tongue must make closure). See that the point of the tongue lies against the lower front teeth. While expelling breath through his nose, have student occlude his nostrils quickly with his thumb and forefinger, forcing the air to separate the velum and back of the tongue. Associate with written "k"; repeat.

10. Have the student lie on his back, relaxed (in this position the velum and

back of the tongue are very close together). Have student breathe through his slightly opened mouth and attempt **k** explosion. *Note:* production will occur far back on the velum and should later be brought forward.

11. Develop the imploded **k** after the imploded-exploded production is accomplished. Demonstrate with techniques similar to those suggested for the sound **p**.

12. If necessary, place teacher's thumb and forefinger on student's throat just under back of the tongue; press upward and forward, then move down quickly. Demonstrate explosion on teacher's production and ask student to attempt the same using his own thumb and forefinger on his throat.

Common Errors and Suggestions for Improvement

1. Excess or insufficient pressure on explosion of breath: Demonstrate as with **p** and **t**. Reduce pressure by having student produce a series of rapid **k** sounds (**kkkkkkkkkk**) on one breath, then produce syllables **kee kee kee kee kee** on another single breath.

2. Lack of closure for stop: Demonstrate by analogy with **p** and **t**. Have student produce series of **ptk** (**ptkptkptkptkptk**) on a single breath. Demonstrate difference between steady breath and sudden explosion with strip of paper or other visual aid. Redevelop in syllables following **ng**: extend **ng** and stop with breath (whispered) explosion. Use visual aids as needed. If **k** closure is accomplished in syllables, tell student to make **ng** without voice and then produce **k** at the end of the syllable.

3. Closure made too far back on velum and tongue: With diagrams compare correct and incorrect placement. Have student keep front of tongue against lower front teeth while producing **k**. Practice **k** in syllables with **ee** and other vowels with forward tongue placement.

*4. Substitution of **g** for **k**, a sonant for surd error:* Write "g" and cross out to make student aware of nature of error. Demonstrate tactile difference as with **b** for **p**, and **d** for **t**. Extend duration of exploded **k** as with **p** and **t**.

5. Mouth too far open: Redevelop, demonstrating that the jaw does not drop on production. Use mirror or, if necessary, place hand under student's jaw on production of a series of **kkkkkkkkkk**. Develop in association with vowel **ee**; use exercises such as **eekee, eekee, eekee,** using a mirror to show that the mouth opening is very slight. Place a pencil or tongue blade between the teeth and have student produce **k** without letting go of object.

6. Explosion made as glottal stop: Redevelop by analogy from **p** and **t**, moving back from **p** to **t** to **k**, and showing place of production by exaggerating if necessary. Redevelop by having student make explosion with closure made by back of tongue on alveolar ridge; gradually move tongue closure back in mouth until a good **k** is produced. Redevelop using development procedure #9, above.

KEY WORDS: **fan, leaf, coffee**

f   /f/   f
SPELLINGS: f, ff, ph, -gh(rough)

Production *(labio-dental breath fricative)*

No voice, nasopharyngeal port closes, the lower lip approximates the upper front teeth, breath is continuously emitted between the teeth and lower lip as audible friction.

Internal Feedback Information

TACTILE: Lower lip lightly touches upper front teeth, friction of restricted breath flow across lower lip.

KINESTHETIC: Lower lip moves upward to approximate upper front teeth.

Sensory Instructional Possibilities

TACTILE: Steady breath flow on skin of the hand.

VISUAL: Approximation of lower lip and upper front teeth can be seen easily. Steady breath flow shown by movement of feather, flame, paper.

Suggestions for Development

1. Imitate from teacher's model; *avoid* excessive pressure on production. Use mirror, if necessary.

2. Demonstrate emission of steady breath with feather, strip of paper, or other visual aid; *avoid* excessive breath pressure or sudden emission.

3. Have student blow, press his lower lip gently upward to approximate the upper front teeth; associate with written "f".

Common Errors and Suggestions for Improvement

1. *Excess force of expelled breath:* Demonstrate that cheeks are not puffed out in producing **f**. Use visual aids to demonstrate difference between appro-

priate and excess breath pressure. Have student produce and extend **f** on a single breath (but do not let student take a deep breath). Draw line after written "f" to show duration of student's production: "f____." Practice extending duration until the force of breath is reduced, then practice a short production, isolated and in syllables **fa(r), fee, foo, faw.**

2. *Excess pressure on contact of lower lip and upper teeth:* Have student produce a rapid series of syllables **fa(r) fa(r) fa(r) fa(r)** on a single breath. Demonstrate degree of pressure by approximating student's index fingers one on top of the other; demonstrate undesirable pressure.

3. *Insufficient breath flow:* Use visual aids or student's hand to demonstrate breath flow. If caused by escape of breath through wide spaces between the teeth, have student approximate the inner surface of the lower lip with the edges and front surface of the teeth. If caused by excess pressure on contact of lower lip and upper teeth, use procedure #2 above.

4. *Substitution of* **v** *for* **f**, *a sonant for surd error:* Write "v" and then cross it out to make student aware of nature of error. Demonstrate the tactile difference by having student feel breath emission on **f** and voice vibration on **v**. Demonstrate greater duration of **f** than **v** by drawing a line to extend the **f:** "f____."

5. *A stop plosive given in place of the fricative:* The student may produce either a **p** sound or a labio-dental stop plosive in place of the fricative **f**. Compare visually, using a mirror if needed. With a strip of paper or other visual aid, show continuing nature of fricative compared to a plosive.

6. *Insertion of* **h**-*like sound after final* **f**, *or between* **f** *and another breath consonant (sof* **h** *t):* Error on final **f** occurs because breath continues after **f** position is released. Practice **f** in final position of syllables **a(r)f, eef, oof,** demonstrating with feather and mirror that breath emission ends before **f** position is released. Contrast inappropriate release to **h**-like sound. With **f** followed by breath stops (**p, t, k**) or affricate **ch**, have student practice terminating the fricative with the stop. With **f** followed by **t**, have student take position for **t**, then produce **ft** blend. Practice in syllables **a(r)ft eft ooft.** With **f** followed by other breath fricatives (*half sole*), practice combinations in blended bisyllables **-afsa- awfsaw eefsee.**

7. *Insertion of natural vowel* -**u**- *between* **f** *and following voiced consonant:* With **f** followed by **r** or **l**, have student take tongue position for **r** or **l** before producing **f**. With **f** followed by voiced stop, have student practice terminating the fricative with the stop (*life belt*). With **f** followed by other voiced consonants or vowels, practice coarticulation in blended syllables.

$\overset{1}{\text{th}}$ /θ/   th

Production *(lingua-dental breath fricative)*

No voice, nasopharyngeal port closes, the tip of the tongue (spread wide and thin) approximates the edge of the upper front teeth, breath is continuously emitted between the front teeth and tongue with audible friction.

Internal Feedback Information

TACTILE: Tongue lightly touches upper front teeth, friction of restricted breath flow across tongue.

KINESTHETIC: Tongue tip moves forward slightly.

Sensory Instructional Possibilities

TACTILE: Steady breath flow on skin of the hand.

VISUAL: Tip of the tongue approximating upper front teeth can be seen through the slightly open front teeth. Steady breath flow shown by movement of feather, flame, paper.

Suggestions for Development

1. Imitate from teacher's model: *avoid* excessive pressure on production. Use mirror if necessary.

2. Demonstrate emission of steady breath with feather, strip of paper, or other visual aid: *avoid* sudden emission of breath.

3. Demonstrate manner of production by analogy to **f.**

4. If necessary, demonstrate place of production by slowly giving a visual exaggeration of the formation: with the teacher's mouth wide open, protrude the tongue, spread it wide and thin, then slowly withdraw it toward position for **th** and produce the sound.

5. If the student is not able to develop **th** otherwise, have him produce it with the tongue protruded between the teeth for improved tactile-kinesthetic feedback. Then have him produce the **th** with the tongue gradually farther back.

Common Errors and Suggestions for Improvement

1. Excess pressure on contact of tongue and upper front teeth: Have student produce the rapid series of syllables $\overset{1}{\text{tha}}$(r) $\overset{1}{\text{tha}}$(r) $\overset{1}{\text{tha}}$(r) $\overset{1}{\text{tha}}$(r) or $\overset{1}{\text{thee}}$ $\overset{1}{\text{thee}}$ $\overset{1}{\text{thee}}$ $\overset{1}{\text{thee}}$ on a single breath. Demonstrate degree of pressure by approximating student's hands or index fingers one on top of the other; compare with undesirable pressure. Place student's fingertip between teacher's upper front teeth and tongue, and demonstrate appropriate pressure with teacher's tongue against student's fingertip.

2. Excess force on expelled breath: Demonstrate as with **f** sound.

3. Substitution of $\overset{2}{\text{th}}$ *for* **th,** *a sonant for surd error:* Write "th" and then cross out to make student aware of nature of error. Demonstrate tactile difference as with **f.**

4. Tip of tongue protruding too far: Redevelop from imitation, using mirror if necessary.

5. Breath escapes from sides of tongue into cheek cavity: Give visual demonstration of the tongue flat and broad, making contact with molars on side. Show with mirror that cheeks are not puffed out on production. Use diagram to show frontal escape of breath. If necessary, gently press student's cheeks inward on production of $\overset{1}{\text{th}}$. If caused by excess breath pressure or excess pressure of tongue contact on front teeth, demonstrate appropriate force as described above.

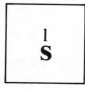

$\overset{1}{\text{s}}$ /s/   s

KEY WORDS: see, makes, upset

SPELLINGS: s, ss, c (e, i, y),

ps-, sc(e, i, y)

Production *(lingua-alveolar breath fricative)*

No voice, nasopharyngeal port closes, the tip of the tongue approximates the alveolar ridge, breath is continuously directed through the narrow aperture between the alveolar ridge and the grooved tip of the tongue against the closely approximated front teeth with audible friction.

Alternate formation: No voice, nasopharyngeal port closes, the tip of the tongue is placed *against the lower front teeth,* the blade of the tongue is elevated to approximate the alveolar ridge and is grooved to form a narrow aperture through which breath is continuously directed against the closely approximated front teeth with audible friction. The essence of s̍ is the forcing of a constricted breath stream against the approximated front teeth; either formation will accomplish this. Both formations are used by normal speakers. Either formation can yield an acceptable s̍ for deaf speakers. Some teachers believe the alternate formation impedes coarticulation with surrounding phonemes. Others find the superior tactile feedback from the tongue tip against the lower front teeth in the alternate formation helpful in developing and maintaining s̍.

Internal Feedback Information

TACTILE: Friction of restricted breath flow across tongue and alveolar ridge. Tip of tongue touches lower front teeth in alternate formation.

KINESTHETIC: Very little feedback from grooving and raising tongue. Because of limited internal feedback information, this is one of the first speech sounds to be affected by hearing loss and is one of the most difficult for deaf persons to monitor.

Sensory Instructional Possibilities

TACTILE: Steady breath flow on skin of hand.

VISUAL: Steady breath flow by movement of feather, flame, paper. Narrow aperture between lower and upper front teeth may be shown with a mirror.

Suggestions for Development

1. Demonstrate manner of production by analogy from **f** and **th̍**.

2. Develop in association with **th̍**. Beginning with the **th̍** position, produce friction gradually withdrawing tongue and approximating front teeth toward s̍ production. Show by diagram that tongue tip moves up toward alveolar ridge as it is withdrawn.

3. Demonstrate emission of steady breath with feather, strip of paper, or other visual aid.

4. Demonstrate place of production by slowly giving a visual exaggeration of formation: with teacher's mouth open wide, show the tongue grooved in the center, then elevated toward the alveolar ridge; slowly narrow mouth opening (keeping tongue in place) toward normal position and produce s̍.

5. Develop in association with **f.** While the student produces a prolonged **f,** pull down his lower lip with two fingers; s̍ may result as student tries to maintain restriction of breath flow with his tongue.

6. Develop in association with **th:** insert a tongue blade between his upper teeth and tongue and gently push tongue back.

7. For alternate formation, demonstrate place of production by slowly giving a visual exaggeration of formation: with teacher's mouth open wide, show the tongue tip behind the lower front teeth and grooved at the center; slowly narrow mouth opening (keeping tongue in place) toward normal position and produce $\overset{1}{s}$.

8. For alternate formation, develop in association with **ee.** Maintaining position for **ee,** giving a whispered production which can be felt on back of the hand. Show the student that the tongue is grooved centrally and that the front approximates the alveolar ridge.

9. Manipulate for appropriate lingua-alveolar openings by inserting a dull pencil point or other slender rounded object between the tongue and alveolar ridge. For the tongue-up $\overset{1}{s}$, begin with the position for **n.** For tongue-down $\overset{1}{s}$, begin with **ee.**

Common Errors and Suggestions for Improvement

1. Inadequate constriction of breath stream directed against teeth: Redevelop, taking care to show grooving of tongue and proximity of tongue to front teeth. Use a diagram to show position if necessary. Demonstrate with feather, strip of paper, or other visual aid that escape of breath is limited to the area of the central incisors and is directed primarily downward on production of an acceptable $\overset{1}{s}$. Compare to diffuse escape of air for unacceptable production. Use mirror for student to imitate acceptable production.

2. Insertion of **t** *either before or after* $\overset{1}{s}$ *production:* In order to achieve better tactile feedback, some deaf speakers may make lingua-alveolar or linguadental closure perceived by the listener as a **t** sound. Write "t" in the position in which it is inserted and cross it out. If **t** is inserted between $\overset{1}{s}$ and the following vowel, it may help to write the word with a faintly written "h" following the $\overset{1}{s}$ to indicate continued breath.

3. Insufficient breath flow: The tongue may be tightly pressed against palate, alveolar ridge or teeth, not permitting a channel for breath. Redevelop showing manner of production by analogy with a series of **f,** then **th,** then $\overset{1}{s}$. Press midline of student's tongue with pencil or other rounded object to show a grooved central passage for air flow.

4. A sound close to **sh** *is produced:* This may be caused by positioning the tongue too far back so that breath flow is diffused. Show student that the tongue approximates the alveolar ridge. If the sound is the result of insufficient pressure of the sides of the tongue closing against the back teeth, have the student raise his jaw slightly for better closure. Pressing upward on both of the student's cheeks may raise the sides of the tongue sufficiently. If necessary, a tongue depressor may be inserted under the sides of the tongue, gently pressing upward to close against the teeth.

5. *Omission of s, especially in final positions of words:* One of the most common and universal errors in the speech of deaf persons, for apparently the s is highly dependent on auditory feedback. Frequently what appears to be an s omission is inadequate pressure on production so that friction is not audible. Demonstrate increased pressure on production, using visual aids. Practice s production in connected words, underlining all s sounds in a written text to be read. Constant reminders with rewards for correct s production. Coordinated school-home effort to emphasize s production in all connected speech. If omission continues, the alternate production (tongue-down or tongue-up) may be developed.

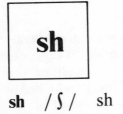

sh   / ʃ /   sh

KEY WORDS: **sh**e, fi**sh**, sun**sh**ine
SPELLINGS: sh, -t(ion), -c(ious)
          ch-(chic), s(sure),
          ch(machine),
          c(ocean),
          -ss-(tissue)

Production *(lingua-palatal breath fricative)*

No voice, nasopharyngeal port closes, the sides of the tongue are against the upper molars, the broad front surface of the tongue is raised toward the alveolar ridge and palate forming a central aperture slightly broader and farther back than for s. Lips are protruded and slightly rounded (approximate lip formation for vowel oo) to direct the breath stream through and against the slightly open front teeth as audible friction.

Internal Feedback Information

TACTILE: Friction of restricted breath flow across tongue, palate, and alveolar ridge.

KINESTHETIC: Some feedback from grooving and raising the tongue. Rounding and protruding of lips.

Sensory Instructional Possibilities

TACTILE: Steady breath flow on skin of the hand.

VISUAL: Rounding and protruding lips seen with mirror. Steady breath flow shown by movement of feather, flame, paper.

Suggestions for Development

1. Imitate from teacher's model; *avoid* excessive pressure on production. Use mirror, if necessary, to show protruded lips and slight opening of teeth.

2. Demonstrate emission of steady breath with feeling on the back of hand, or with a feather, strip of paper, or other visual aid; *avoid* sudden emission of breath.

3. Demonstrate manner of production by analogy from **th** and **s**. Show student that the tongue is moved successively back from **th** to **s** to **sh** production.

4. Demonstrate place of production by slowly giving a visual exaggeration of the formation: with the teacher's mouth open wide, show the broad front of the tongue well behind the lower front teeth, slowly narrow mouth opening (keeping tongue in place) toward normal position, protrude and round the lips; produce **sh**. Have student attempt to imitate this production using a mirror, if necessary.

5. Develop in association with **ee**. Maintaining the mouth opening position for **ee,** protrude the lips and give a whispered production. Have the student feel the emission of breath on his hand. Similarly, develop in association with **r,** giving a whispered production with the lips rounded and protruded, and maintaining the tongue position for **r.**

6. Manipulate for appropriate position by using the following steps for production: have the student imitate the teacher opening the mouth (about two fingers' space between the teeth), protrude and point the tongue straight out, have the student place the tip of his index finger against the point of his tongue, have the student slowly push the point of his tongue back into the mouth well behind the lower front teeth (being careful not to let the tongue tip curl upward) until the broad front of the tongue is observed, have student slowly protrude his lips while the index finger maintains the broad front of the tongue in place. Close teeth gently on the index finger with upper and lower front teeth partly showing (not covered by lips), produce the **sh** approximation with the finger still holding the tongue in place. Remove the finger (keeping the tongue in place) and produce **sh** again. Teeth opening may be reduced further for improved production. Repeat until student has produced **sh**. Use a mirror if necessary.

7. Manipulate in association with the **th** sound. While the student produces an extended **th,** gently push the lip of the tongue back inside the mouth well

behind the lower front teeth. When an approximation of **sh** is reached, have the student attempt pulling back without help of the finger. Have student protrude and slightly round the lips on production.

Common Errors and Suggestions for Improvement

1. Inadequate constriction of the breath stream: Redevelop, taking care to show by teacher example or diagrams that the tongue is raised high in the mouth, the sides of the tongue are against the upper molars directing the flow of breath centrally, and the teeth are only slightly open. Demonstrate by feeling on the hand, or by using a feather, strip of paper, or other visual aids, that the flow of breath is reduced. Compare to excessive breath emission. Demonstrate constriction of breath by analogy from **t̪h** and **s̪**.

2. Excessive constriction of the breath stream: To achieve feedback, the student may seek to close the tongue point against the alveolar ridge or palate, causing lateral emission of breath, or he may press it against the lower front teeth, causing an **s̪**-like sound. Redevelop, using the procedures in development technique #6, above, emphasizing that the broad front of the tongue is well behind the lower front teeth. Redevelop, taking care to have student feel the sides of the tongue against the upper molars. If necessary, have the student close the lower molars gently up against the sides of the tongue, also, so that the flattened sides of the tongue are sandwiched between the upper and lower molars. In this position the steady emission of breath will not permit the tongue tip to close against the alveolar ridge or palate.

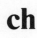

KEY WORDS: **ch**air, su**ch**, tea**ch**er
SPELLINGS: ch, -tch, -t(ure),
-t(ion)

ch /tʃ/ ch

Production *(lingua-alveolar, lingua-palatal breath affricate)*

No voice, nasopharyngeal port closes, the sides of the tongue are against the upper molars, lips are protruded and slightly rounded (as for **sh**), the front of the tongue closes just behind the alveolar ridge; air held and compressed in the oral cavity is exploded as audible breath through the aperture between the alveolar ridge and tongue, and against the slightly open front teeth as audible friction.

The position is essentially that for the **sh** except that, instead of the steady flow of breath for friction, breath is imploded and exploded by the tongue closure slightly farther back on the alveolar ridge than for the **t** sound, and released more slowly but with greater pressure than for the **t**. This phoneme is produced with a single impulse of breath, even though it includes components of both the **t** and the **sh** sounds.

Internal Feedback Information

TACTILE: Point of the tongue touches the alveolar ridge; exploded air is felt across the tongue, palate, and alveolar ridge.

KINESTHETIC: Movement of tongue slightly upward to alveolar ridge, grooving of tongue on release of compressed air. Rounding and protruding of lips.

Sensory Instructional Possibilities

TACTILE: Exploded air on skin of the hand.

VISUAL: Rounding and protruding of lips seen with mirror. Explosion of air shown by movement of feather, flame, paper strip.

Suggestions for Development

Note: the **ch** is best developed after the **sh** can be produced well.

1. Imitate from teacher's model. Let student feel explosion of breath on back of his hand. *Avoid* excessive dropping of jaw on production.

2. Develop by analogy from **sh**. Have the student produce **sh** and write it on the chalk board. Now show the student the closure of the tongue against the alveolar ridge and produce **ch,** letting him feel the explosion of breath.

3. Demonstrate place of production by slowly giving a visual exaggeration of the formation: with the teacher's mouth open wide, show the tip of the tongue just behind the alveolar ridge, slowly narrow mouth opening toward normal position, protrude and round the lips; produce **ch** with a slight jaw dropping.

4. Develop in association with **sh**. Have the student produce an extended **sh** with interruptions of the continued breath flow for tongue closure as in **t**. Have the student imitate the teacher's pattern. The pattern may be represented by writing the "sh" on the chalk board with a tail interrupted as follows: "sh____/ /____/ /____/ /____," or as "sh____t____t____t," writing the "t" very small. When the **ch** is produced in these patterns, have the student produce it in isolation and with vowel sounds.

5. Develop by analogy from **t** and **sh**. Have the student produce the following series: **t sh tsh ch**. Demonstrate that the **ch** is made on a single breath impulse as compared to the **tsh** combination.

Common Errors and Suggestions for Improvement

1. Inadequate friction on production: Redevelop by analogy from **sh**. Have the student produce **sh** and write it on the chalk board. Show the student closure of the tongue against the alveolar ridge and produce **ch,** letting him feel the explosion of breath. Redevelop in association with **sh**. Follow suggested technique #4 for development of **ch**.

2. Failure to make the plosive tongue closure: The student may produce the **sh** sound in substitution for **ch,** or he may produce a short burst of breath by glottal closure and release. Redevelop place of production by slowly giving a visual exaggeration of the formation; follow suggested technique #3 for development. Emphasize position of tongue for closure and release. Have student imitate each step, using mirror if necessary, making certain that he accomplishes tongue closure on the alveolar ridge. Exaggerate the plosive manner of production, dropping jaw and letting student feel sudden explosion of breath on his hand. When student makes satisfactory production, demonstrate that **ch** should be produced without dropping the jaw. Demonstrate plosive manner of production by analogy; produce a series as follows: **p t k ch p t k ch.** Demonstrate plosive action by pressing the fingers of one hand on the palm of the other, and then release them suddenly.

3. Production of two breath impulses as in **t** *and* **sh** *combination:* Redevelop as **ch** on a single breath impulse. Contrast the **tsh** combination with the single impulse **ch,** letting student feel the difference on his hand. Write "tsh" and "ch" on the chalk board, comparing the two and then crossing out the "tsh." Write the "tsh" combination on the chalk board with the "t" written very small.

4. Extended duration of fricative finish: Practice repeated short productions of **ch** on a single breath (**ch ch ch ch ch ch**).

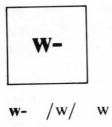

w-   /w/   w

Production *(bilabial voiced resonant)*

With voice, the nasopharyngeal port closes, the lips are rounded and slightly protruded. Lip protrusion is not so great as for **oo;** lip aperture is smaller than for o͡o. The **w-** is always released into a vowel; taking the lip rounded position described above, the **w-** is very brief, rapidly gliding into the formation of the following vowel.

Internal Feedback Information

TACTILE: Voicing may be felt.

KINESTHETIC: Rounding and protruding of lips.

AUDITORY: May be heard in a syllable but duration is very short.

Sensory Instructional Possibilities

TACTILE: Vibration of voicing with hand on lips or cheeks.

VISUAL: Rounding and protruding of lips.

Suggestions for Development

1. Develop **w-** in syllables using a wide variety of vowels; emphasize the relatively short duration of the **w-** in relation to the following vowel.

2. Imitate from teacher's model. Use mirror, if necessary. Show student that lip protrusion is not so great as for o͡o.

3. With student and teacher seated side-by-side, show in a mirror the degree of rounding and protrusion of the lips.

4. Develop by analogy to **wh.** Show student by tactile impression that breath is not expelled and that voice vibration is present.

5. Develop by analogy to o͡o. By underlining, show the student that **w-** is shorter than o͡o as follows: "wo͡o."

6. If the student has difficulty rounding the lips, trace a circle around his lips with the teacher's index fingertip. If the lips are not sufficiently protruded, the circle tracing finger may be held just beyond the lips, with teacher urging the student to touch her finger with his lips.

7. If necessary, manipulate the lips with teacher's thumb and index finger, pressing the corners of the mouth inward toward the rounded position.

Common Errors and Suggestions for Improvement

1. Duration too great (similar to duration of o͡o*):* By underlining, show student that **w-** is shorter than o͡o, as in development suggestion #5 above. Write syllables with **w-**; underline the vowel and only the last part of the **w-** as follows: "w- ee."

2. Produced with audible breath friction (usually associated with extended duration); may be heard as **wh:** Reduce duration, as described above. Demonstrate the lack of breath flow by tactile impression on student's hand.

3. *Exaggerated rounding of the lips:* Redevelop in syllables using a narrow but not rounded lip opening.

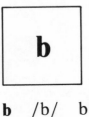

b /b/ b

KEY WORDS: **b**oy, ca**b**, ra**bb**it
SPELLINGS: b, bb

Production *(bilabial voiced stop)*

IMPLOSION: With voice, nasopharyngeal port closes, lips close, air is held and compressed briefly in the oral cavity while voicing continues.

EXPLOSION: Lips, held together with less pressure and for shorter duration than for **p,** are opened; voicing continues.

In connected speech, "closure" and "release" more accurately describe the force of action for producing **b** than do "implosion" and "explosion." The **b** is closed but not released with voicing as the final sound of an utterance or immediately before a breath consonant (*lab, coat*). As the initial sound of an utterance or immediately following a breath consonant, voicing begins with the lips closed and the **b** is released into the following voiced sound. As a sound between two voiced sounds, **b** is a brief closure and release with voicing continuing. The sound **b** cannot be produced in isolation; it is often identified as a phoneme in a syllable preceding the natural vowel, as in **bu-.**

Internal Feedback Information

TACTILE: Lips touch with closure, voicing may be felt.

KINESTHETIC: Lips close lightly with less force than on **p.**

AUDITORY: In a syllable with a vowel, can be heard but duration is very brief.

Sensory Instructional Possibilities

TACTILE: Vibration of voicing with hand on lips or cheeks.

VISUAL: Lip closure and opening seen easily.

Suggestions for Development

1. Imitate from teacher's model in syllables; *avoid* dropping jaw and produc-

ing excess pressure. Produce a series of **b** closures with continuing voice (**bubububububu-**).

2. Have student use mirror to monitor his production if he cannot imitate the teacher's pattern otherwise.

3. If necessary, develop **b** by analogy to **p,** demonstrating the absence of explosion for **b** and the presence of voicing. *Avoid* producing the sounds **b** and **p** with equal force.

4. Develop the imploded (unreleased) **b** after the released production is accomplished. Imitate from teacher's model of vowel interrupted by lip closure as in **-ub;** use a series of **-ubububububub** and contrast with **bubububububu-** where final **b** is released.

5. If necessary, demonstrate that the final **b** is not released by teacher placing her finger over her lips to apparently prevent release. The unreleased sound may be written "**-b**" compared to the released "**b-.**"

Common Errors and Suggestions for Improvement

1. Excess pressure on release: Demonstrate reduced pressure by tactile impression of absence of breath on student's hand. Contrast with excess breath explosion. Have the student produce a series of relaxed syllables (**bubububububububu-**) on the same breath.

*2. Substitution of **p** for **b,** a surd for sonant error:* Write "p" and cross it out to make student aware of the nature of his error. Demonstrate the tactile difference by having student feel voice vibration on **b** and explosion of breath on **p.** Instruct student to reduce pressure on release; write "b" faintly or with dotted writing to show reduced pressure on production. Instruct student to make **b** of shorter duration or say it faster; contrast with **p** duration using written symbols: "b" vs. "p   ."

*3. Substitution of **m** for **b,** a nasal error:* With breathy emission, show with strip of paper or other visual aid. Demonstrate inappropriate nasal emission by having student feel vibration on his nose with **m** but not with **b.** Have student produce a series of syllables on a single breath (**bubububububu-**), interrupting the series by occluding the student's nostrils. Have student attempt the series occluding his own nostrils, then without occlusion.

*4. Release of final **b** and **b** before voiced consonants:* Redevelop the unreleased **b** in syllables (**-ubububububub**). If necessary, place finger over the lips at conclusion of the series to prevent release. With vowel following **b,** practice production of coarticulated **b** and vowel in a series (**beebeebeebeebeebee**), (**bawbawbawbawbawbaw**) using mirror, if needed. With **l** or **r** following **b,** practice production for coarticulation by having student first take the tongue position for **l** or **r**, then produce the **b** in combination with **l** or **r** and a vowel, as in **bloo, bla(r), blee,** or **broo, bra(r), bree.** For timing, duration of syllable **bloo** should be not much (if at all) longer than **boo;** have student practice series of syllables (**boo boo boo bloo bloo bloo boo boo boo**), attempting the same duration on each syllable. Repeat with other vowels.

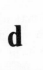

d   /d/   d

KEY WORDS: **d**ay, mu**d**, la**dd**er
SPELLINGS: d, dd

Production *(lingua-alveolar voiced stop)*

IMPLOSION: With voice, nasopharyngeal port closes, point of the tongue closes against alveolar ridge and side of tongue against molars, air is held and compressed briefly in the oral cavity while voicing continues.

EXPLOSION: Closure of point of tongue on alveolar ridge (held with less pressure for shorter duration than for **t**) is released; voicing continues.

In connected speech, "closure" and "release" more accurately describe the force of action for producing **d** than do "implosion" and "explosion." The **d** is closed but not released with voicing as the final sound of an utterance (*mud, sad*) or immediately before a breath consonant (*bedtime*). As the initial sound of an utterance or immediately following a breath consonant, voicing begins with the lingua-alveolar closure and the **d** is released into the following voiced sound. Between two voiced sounds, **d** is a brief closure and release with continued voicing. The sound **d** (like **b**) cannot be produced in isolation; it is usually identified as a phoneme in a syllable preceding the natural vowel, as in **du-.**

Internal Feedback Information

TACTILE: Point of the tongue touches the alveolar ridge, voicing may be felt.

KINESTHETIC: Movement of tongue slightly upward to alveolar ridge, closure lighter than for **t.**

AUDITORY: In a syllable with a vowel can be heard but duration is very brief.

Sensory Instructional Possibilities

TACTILE: Vibration of voicing with hand on lips or cheeks.

VISUAL: Raised tongue point seen through the slightly separated teeth.

Suggestions for Development

1. Imitate from teacher's model in syllables; *avoid* dropping jaw and producing excess pressure. Produce a series of **d** closures with continuing voice (**dudududududu-**).

2. Have student use mirror to monitor his productions, if necessary.

3. If necessary, develop **d** by analogy to **t,** demonstrating the absence of explosion for **d** and the presence of voicing. *Avoid* producing the sounds **d** and **t** with equal force.

4. Develop the imploded (unreleased) **d** after the released production is accomplished. Imitate from teacher's model of vowel interrupted by lingua-alveolar closure as in **-ud;** use a series such as **-ududududud;** contrast **dududududu-** where the final **d** is released.

5. If necessary, demonstrate that final **d** is not released by teacher's placing her finger over her lips to prevent release. The unreleased sound may be written "-d" compared to released "d-."

Common Errors and Suggestions for Improvement

1. Excess pressure on release: Demonstrate reduced pressure by tactile impression of absence of breath on student's hand. Contrast with excess breath explosion. Have the student produce a series of relaxed syllables (**dudududududu-**) on the same breath.

*2. Substitution of **t** for **d**, a surd for sonant error:* Write "t" and cross it out to make student aware of the nature of his error. Demonstrate the tactile difference by having student feel voice vibration on **d** and explosion of breath on **t.** Instruct student to reduce pressure on release; write "d" faintly or with dotted writing to show reduced pressure on production. Instruct student to make **d** of shorter duration or say it faster; contrast with **t** duration using written symbols: "d___" vs. "t_____."

*3. Substitution of **n** for **d**, a nasal error:* With breathy emission of **n,** demonstrate inappropriate nasal emission with strip of paper or other visual aid. Demonstrate inappropriate nasal emission by having student feel vibration on his nose with **n** but not with **d.** Have student produce a series of syllables on a single breath (**dududududu-**), interrupting the series by occluding the student's nostrils. Have student attempt the series occluding his own nostrils, then without occlusion.

*4. Release of final **d** and **d** before voiced consonants:* Redevelop the unreleased **d** in syllables (**-udududududud**). If necessary, place hand over the mouth opening at conclusion of the series to prohibit release. With vowel following **d,** practice production of coarticulation in a syllable series (**deedeedeedee- deedee**), using mirror, if needed; see that jaw does not move appreciably with syllables.

With lingua-alveolar consonants **n** or **t** following **d,** practice coarticulation on syllables without moving tongue position *(had not, had to).* With lingua-al- veolar **l** following **d,** practice keeping tongue tip on alveolar ridge, narrowing tongue for lateral emission *(badly, would let).* With lingua-alveolar fricatives $\overset{1}{s}$ and **z** following **d,** practice coarticulation with only slight movement of tongue for release into the fricative *(could see, good zoo).* With lingua-dental $\overset{2}{th}$ following **d** *(had the, hid them),* produce the **d** with closure forward on the back of the upper front teeth opening slightly for release into the fricative with only slight tongue protrusion for the $\overset{2}{th}$. For the **dr-** blend, practice mak- ing the sound in syllables, moving the tongue back on the alveolar ridge as the **d** is being formed, releasing the closure into the **r.**

5. *Too wide a mouth opening:* Have the student produce a series of syl- lables **dee dee dee** and **eed eed eed,** observing his productions in a mirror; there should be no movement of the jaw. The student may hold a pencil eraser between his teeth while producing these syllables to assure that the jaw does not drop.

g

g /g/ g

KEY WORDS: **go, log, begged**
SPELLINGS: g, gg

Production *(lingua-velar voiced stop)*

IMPLOSION: With voice, nasopharyngeal port closes, back of the tongue closes against front portion of velum or back portion of palate, air is held and com- pressed briefly in the back of the oral cavity while voicing continues. *Note:* the point of contact on the velum-palate changes with surrounding vowels.

EXPLOSION: Closure of back of tongue and velum-palate—held together with less pressure and for shorter duration than the **k**—is released; voicing contin- ues.

In connected speech, "closure" and "release" more accurately describe the force of action for producing **g** than do "implosion" and "explosion." The **g** is closed but not released with voicing as the final sound of an utterance (*bag, rag*) or immediately before a breath consonant (*rag time*). As the initial sound of an utterance or immediately following a breath consonant, voicing begins with the lingua-velar closure and the **g** is released into the following voiced sound. As a sound between two voiced sounds, **g** is a brief closure and is released with continued voicing.

Internal Feedback Information

TACTILE: Closure of back of tongue on velum or palate gives little information; voicing may be felt.

KINESTHETIC: Raising of back of tongue to close against velum or palate gives little information; closure lighter than for **k**.

AUDITORY: In syllable with a vowel, can be heard but duration is very brief.

Sensory Instructional Possibilities

TACTILE: Vibration of voicing with hand on lips, cheeks, or throat.

VISUAL: Place of production visible only with exaggerated mouth opening.

Suggestions for Development

1. Imitate from teacher's model in syllables; *avoid* dropping jaw and producing excess pressure. Produce a series of **g** closures with continuing voice (**gugugugugugu-**).

2. Demonstrate manner of production by analogy from **b** and **d**. If necessary to demonstrate place of production as well as manner, show the analogy to the **k** sound. Produce the series **p t k,** then **b d g.**

3. Demonstrate place of production by slowly giving a visual exaggeration of the formation as with **k.**

4. Demonstrate manner and place of production by giving a visually exaggerated step-by-step production as with **k.**

5. Develop **g** in association with the **ee** vowel, a position in which the tongue is very close to the velum-palate, **eeg** or **gee**. Develop **g** in association with **ng,** using such syllables as **eeng g.**

6. While the student attempts to produce **d,** hold tip of his tongue down (with finger or tongue blade) behind the lower front teeth (do not let the back of the tongue move forward). Associate the sound he releases with written "g." After several repetitions with the teacher or student holding down the tip of the tongue, have the student attempt the production without this aid.

7. Have the student produce and extend **ng.** While this is being produced have student occlude his nostrils quickly with thumb and forefinger while voicing continues, forcing a separation of the velum and back of the tongue. Associate the resulting release sound with the written "g."

8. Develop the imploded (unreleased) **g** after the released production is accomplished. Demonstrate the techniques similar to those for **b** and **d.**

Common Errors and Suggestions for Improvement

1. Excess pressure on release: Demonstrate reduced pressure by tactile impression of absence of breath on student's hand. Contrast with excess breath explosion. Have student produce a relaxed series of syllables (**gugugugugugu-**) on the same breath. If **b** and **d** have appropriate pressure and release, associate **g** with these sounds in a syllable series of **budugu-budugu-budugu-** on a single breath.

2. Closure made too far back on velum and tongue: With diagrams compare correct and incorrect placement. Have student keep front of tongue against lower front teeth while producing **g.** Practice **g** in syllables with **ee** and other vowels with forward tongue placement.

3. Substitution of **k** *for* **g,** *a surd for sonant error:* Write "k" and cross it out to make student aware of nature of error. Demonstrate tactile difference as with **p** for **b** and **t** for **d.** Instruct student to reduce pressure and duration as with **b** and **d.**

4. Release of final **g** *and of* **g** *before voiced consonants:* Redevelop the unreleased **g** in syllables (**-ugugugugug**). If necessary, place hand over mouth opening at conclusion of the series to prevent release. With a vowel following **g,** practice production of coarticulation in a syllable series of **ga(r), ga(r), ga(r), ga(r);** see that the jaw does not drop on syllable production.

With **k** following **g** in connected speech (*big king*), practice coarticulation on syllables without moving tongue position. With **gr-** and **gl-** blends, practice positioning tongue tip for **r** and **l** sounds before the **g** is produced; release **g** into the **r** or **l.** Then produce syllables such as **gloo, glee, groo.** For timing, duration of syllable **gloo** should be not much (if at all) longer than **goo;** have student practice series of syllables **goo goo goo gloo gloo gloo goo goo goo** attempting the same duration on each syllable.

5. Mouth too far open: Redevelop, demonstrating that the jaw does not drop on production in isolation. Use mirror or, if necessary, place hand over child's jaw on production of a series of **gggggg.** Develop in association with vowel **ee;** use exercises such as **eegee, eegee, eegee** using a mirror to show that the mouth opening is very slight. Place a pencil or tongue blade between the teeth and have student produce **g** without letting go of object.

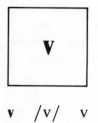

KEY WORDS: vine, give, every
SPELLINGS: v, -f(of),
-ph-(Stephen)

v /v/ v

Production *(labio-dental voiced fricative)*

With voice, nasopharyngeal port closes, the lower lip approximates the upper front teeth, voice is continuously emitted with escape between the teeth and lower lip as combined voice and audible friction. Duration is shorter and produced with less force than for **f.** In termination of an utterance the **v** has a breath finish.

Internal Feedback Information

TACTILE: Lower lip lightly touches upper front teeth, friction of restricted breath flow across lower lip. Voicing may be felt.

KINESTHETIC: Lower lip moves upward to approximate upper front teeth.

AUDITORY: Acoustically weak, and duration is very short.

Sensory Instructional Possibilities

TACTILE: Slight flow of breath on skin of the hand. Vibration of voicing by hand on lips or cheeks.

VISUAL: Approximation of lower lip and upper front teeth can be easily seen.

Suggestions for Development

1. Imitate from teacher's model; *avoid* excessive pressure on production. Use mirror, if necessary.

2. Develop by analogy from **f,** demonstrating the absence of escaping breath flow and the presence of voicing. *Avoid* producing **v** with pressure equal to **f.**

3. Demonstrate vibration of lower lip by having student feel teacher's lip as she produces **v.**

4. Have student produce and extend the vowel **-u-,** press his lower lip gently upward to approximate the upper front teeth; associate with written "v."

Common Errors and Suggestions for Improvement

1. Breath flow insufficient for audible friction: Use visual aids or tactile impression on student's hand to demonstrate breath flow. If caused by escape of breath through side spaces between the teeth, have student approximate the inner surface of the lower lip with the edges and front surface of the teeth. If caused by excess pressure on contact of lower lip and upper teeth, demonstrate degree of pressure by approximating student's index fingers one on top of the other; demonstrate undesirable pressure.

*2. Substitution of **f** for **v**, a surd for sonant error;* Write "f " and then cross it out to make student aware of nature of error. Demonstrate the tactile difference as described for **f**. The **v** may be improved by having the edge of the upper front teeth contact just inside the lower lip, rather than on the top surface of the lower lip as with **f**.

3. Nasal emission of voice: Demonstrate tactile impression of vibration on the lower lip and absence of voice vibration on the nose with **v**. Redevelop by analogy from **f**; have student produce extended **f** blending into extended **v** (**f___v___f___v**) on a single breath.

*4. Release of final **v** with -u- sound.* Voicing continues after **v** is released. Contrast released and unreleased **v**, demonstrating tactile and visual differences. Have student release final **v** sound with a soft breath release. Write as "-vf" with the "f" written faintly.

5. Extended duration: Draw line after "f" to show its duration ("f_____"), compare with **v** drawing a much shorter line ("v__"). Practice a series of short syllables (**veeveeveeveeveevee**) on a single breath.

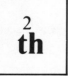

KEY WORDS: **the**, smoo**th**, bo**th**er
SPELLINGS: th-, -th(er),
       -th(s), -th(e)

²**th** /ð/ ~~th~~

Production *(lingua-dental voiced fricative)*

With voice, nasopharyngeal port closes, the tip of the tongue approximates the edge of the upper front teeth, voice is continuously emitted with escape between the front teeth and tongue as combined voice and audible friction.

Duration is shorter and produced with less force than for $\overset{1}{th}$. In termination of an utterance the $\overset{2}{th}$ has a breath finish.

Internal Feedback Information

TACTILE: Tongue lightly touches upper front teeth, friction of restricted breath flow across tongue. Voicing can be felt.

KINESTHETIC: Tongue tip moves forward slightly.

AUDITORY: Acoustically very weak, and duration is very short.

Sensory Instructional Possibilities

TACTILE: Slight flow of breath felt on skin of the hand. Vibration of voicing can be felt by hand on cheeks, or by fingertips on extended tongue tip.

VISUAL: Tip of the tongue approximating upper front teeth can be seen through the slightly open front teeth.

Suggestions for Development

1. Imitate from teacher's model; *avoid* excessive pressure on production. Use mirror, if necessary.

2. Develop by analogy from v for manner of production. Develop by analogy from $\overset{1}{th}$ for place of production; demonstrate absence of escaping breath flow and the presence of voicing for $\overset{2}{th}$. Avoid producing $\overset{2}{th}$ with pressure equal to $\overset{1}{th}$.

3. Demonstrate voice vibration by having the student feel the protruded tip of the teacher's tongue as she produces $\overset{2}{th}$.

4. Have the student produce and extend the vowel -u-, extending his tongue tip beyond the edge of the upper teeth. Gently press his tongue upward against the edge of the upper teeth as voicing continues.

Common Errors and Suggestions for Improvement

1. Substitution of $\overset{1}{th}$ for $\overset{2}{th}$, a surd for sonant error: Write "th" and then cross it out to make student aware of nature of error. Demonstrate the tactile difference of reduced breath flow and presence of voicing on production of $\overset{2}{th}$ compared to $\overset{1}{th}$. The $\overset{2}{th}$ may be improved by having the tip of the tongue approximate the upper front teeth just inside the edge (slightly less tongue protrusion than for $\overset{1}{th}$).

2. Nasal emission of voice: Demonstrate the tactile impression of vibration on the slightly protruded tongue and the absence of voice vibration on the nose with $\overset{2}{th}$. Redevelop by analogy from $\overset{1}{th}$. Gently close off the nostrils, if necessary.

z

KEY WORDS: **z**oo, si**z**e, la**z**y
SPELLINGS: z, s

z /z/ z

Production *(lingua-alveolar voiced fricative)*

With voice, the nasopharyngeal port closes, the tip of the tongue approximates the alveolar ridge, voiced breath is continuously directed through the narrow aperture between the alveolar ridge and the grooved tip of the tongue against the closely approximated front teeth as combined voice and audible friction. Duration is shorter and produced with less force than for **$\overset{1}{s}$.** The initial **z** requires more breath pressure than do the voiced fricatives **v** and **$\overset{2}{th}$.** In termination of an utterance *(run*s*)*, the **z** has a breath finish.

Alternate formation: see description of tongue-down formation for **$\overset{1}{s}$.**

Internal Feedback Information

TACTILE: Slight friction of restricted breath flow across tongue and alveolar ridge. Voicing may be felt.

KINESTHETIC: Very little feedback from grooving and raising the tongue.

AUDITORY: Acoustically weak, and duration is short.

Sensory Instructional Possibilities

TACTILE: Vibration of voicing can be felt by hand under chin near base of the tongue, or by finger tips on teeth. Slight flow of breath on skin of the hand.

VISUAL: Narrow aperture between lower and upper front teeth may be shown with a mirror.

Suggestions for Development

1. Develop by analogy from **$\overset{1}{s}$,** demonstrating the presence of voicing with **z.** Let student feel vibration of teeth and chin. Modify suggestions for developing **$\overset{1}{s}$.**

2. Demonstrate manner of production by analogy from **v** and **$\overset{2}{th}$.** Contrast **v** with **f, $\overset{2}{th}$** with **$\overset{1}{th}$,** then **z** with **$\overset{1}{s}$.**

3. Develop in association with **$\overset{2}{th}$.** Beginning with the **$\overset{2}{th}$** position, produce

voiced friction, gradually withdrawing tongue and approximating front teeth toward **z** production. Show by diagram that the tongue tip moves up toward the alveolar ridge as it is withdrawn.

4. Demonstrate place of production by slowly giving a visual exaggeration of formation: with teacher's mouth wide open, show the tongue grooved in the center then elevated toward the alveolar ridge (tongue tip behind the lower front teeth for alternate formation), slowly narrow mouth opening toward normal position and produce **z**.

5. *Note:* When it is the terminating consonant preceded by a voiced sound (*tabs, goods, bags, knives*), the teacher may choose to develop the **z** as an $\overset{1}{s}$ in order to reduce voicing at the finish.

Common Errors and Suggestions for Improvement

1. Inadequate breath flow on production: Redevelop by analogy from $\overset{1}{s}$, emphasizing the flow of breath on both sounds; exaggerate the breath flow on **z,** if necessary. Relax excessive pressure to permit escape of breath stream if production is inhibited by too much constriction.

2. Inadequate voicing in the production: Redevelop by analogy from **v** and $\overset{2}{th}$. Develop in association with **ee,** producing alternate sounds **z** and **ee** on a single breath (**eezeezeezeezeezeez**).

3. Excessive voicing and duration as a terminating sound: Demonstrate the breath finish by writing the sound as "**z–s**," as in the word *goods.* Point out that the breath finish has diminished pressure by writing the **s** finish small or in dotted lines. The teacher may choose to develop this terminating sound as $\overset{1}{s}$ following voiced sounds. Voicing from the preceding sound will infiltrate the $\overset{1}{s}$ to give the acoustic impression of a final **z** sound.

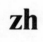

zh /ʒ/ zh

KEY WORDS: measure, vision, usual
SPELLINGS: -s(ion), -s(sure),
-g(e)(loge)

Production *(lingua-palatal voiced fricative)*

With voice, the nasopharyngeal port closes, the sides of the tongue are against the upper molars, the broad front surface of the tongue is raised toward the alveolar ridge and palate forming a central aperture slightly broader and farther back than for $\overset{1}{s}$. Lips are protruded and slightly rounded (approximate lip formation for vowel $\overset{2}{oo}$) to direct the voiced breath stream through and against the slightly open front teeth as combined voice and audible friction.

Internal Feedback Information

TACTILE: Slight friction of restricted breath flow across tongue, palate, and alveolar ridge. Voicing can be felt.

KINESTHETIC: Some feedback from grooving and raising the tongue. Rounding and protruding of lips.

AUDITORY: Acoustically weak, and duration is short.

Sensory Instructional Possibilities

TACTILE: Vibration of voicing can be felt by hand on sides of neck and under chin near the base of the tongue.

VISUAL: Rounding and protruding of lips can be seen with mirror.

Suggestions for Development

Note: this sound does not typically occur in children's early vocabulary.

1. Development by analogy from **sh,** demonstrating the presence of voicing with **zh.**

2. Demonstrate manner of production by analogy from **v,** $\overset{2}{th}$ and **z.** Contrast **f** and **v,** $\overset{1}{th}$ and $\overset{2}{th}$, $\overset{1}{s}$ and **z,** then **sh** and **zh.** Show student that the tongue is moved successively back from $\overset{2}{th}$ to **z** to **zh.**

3. Demonstrate place of production by slowly giving a visual exaggeration of the formation, as with **sh.**

4. Develop in association with **ee.** Maintaining the mouth opening position for **ee,** protrude the lips and produce **zh.** Have the student feel the emission of breath on his hand.

5. Manipulate in association with the $\overset{2}{th}$ sound, as for development of **sh** from $\overset{1}{th}$.

6. As a terminating consonant (*garage*) the **zh** has a breath finish. Demonstrate by writing the sound as "zh__sh." Point out the breath finish has diminished pressure by writing the **sh** finish small or in dotted lines.

Common Errors and Suggestions for Improvement

1. Inadequate breath flow on production: Redevelop by analogy from **sh,** emphasizing the flow of breath on both **sh** and **zh**; exaggerate the breath flow on **zh,** if necessary, letting student feel tactile impression on his hand. Redevelop, taking care to show by teacher example or diagram that the tongue is raised high in the mouth, the sides of the tongue are against the upper molars directing the flow of breath centrally, with a fairly broad aperture.

2. *Inadequate voicing in production:* Redevelop by analogy from **v**, **t͡h**, and **z**.

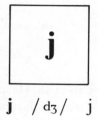

j / dʒ / j

KEY WORDS: **j**am, e**dg**e, enjoy
SPELLINGS: j, -dg(e), -g(e)

Production *(lingua-alveolar/lingua-palatal voiced affricate)*

With voice, the nasopharyngeal port closes, the sides of the tongue are against the upper molars, lips are protruded and slightly rounded (as for **sh**), the front of the tongue closes just behind the alveolar ridge; air held and compressed briefly in the oral cavity is released as breath and voice combined through the aperture between the alveolar ridge and tongue, and against the slightly open front teeth as audible friction. The position is essentially that for the **ch**, except that voicing is involved. It may also be considered a single impulse production of combined **dzh**. The explosion is released with less pressure than for **ch** but with greater force than for **d**. Tongue placement for closure is slightly farther back on the alveolar ridge than for **d**.

Internal Feedback Information

TACTILE: Point of the tongue touches the alveolar ridge. Voicing may be felt; slight friction of restricted breath flow across tongue, palate, and alveolar ridge.

KINESTHETIC: Movement of tongue slightly upward to alveolar ridge, grooving of tongue on release of compressed air. Rounding and protruding of lips.

AUDITORY: In a syllable with a vowel, can be heard but duration is very brief.

Sensory Instructional Possibilities

TACTILE: Vibration of voicing felt by hand under chin near base of the tongue.

VISUAL: Raised tongue point can be seen through the slightly open teeth. Rounding and protruding of lips can be seen with mirror.

Suggestions for Development

Note: the **j** is best developed after the **d** and **ch** can be produced well.

1. Imitate from teacher's model; *avoid* dropping jaw on production.

2. Develop by analogy from **ch,** demonstrating the presence of voicing with **j.**

3. Demonstrate manner of production by analogy from other voiced plosives. Have student produce a series of **b, d, g, j.** Contrast **p** and **b, t** and **d, k** and **g,** and then **ch** and **j.**

4. Develop by analogy from **zh** (if the student can produce a good **zh**), using techniques suggested in developing **ch** by analogy from **sh.**

Common Errors and Suggestions for Improvement

1. Inadequate friction on production: Redevelop by analogy from **zh.** Have the student produce **zh** and write it on the chalk board. Show student closure of the tongue against the alveolar ridge and produce **j,** letting the student feel the explosion of breath.

*2. Production of two voice impulses as in **d** and **zh** combination:* Contrast the **dzh** combination with the single impulse **j,** letting student feel the difference on his hand.

3. Extended vocalization as a terminating consonant: Demonstrate that **j** has a breath finish as a terminating consonant by writing it as "d__sh," writing the "sh" in small letters or dotted lines to show that it is de-emphasized.

m /m/   m

KEY WORDS: **m**eat, tea**m**, ca**m**era
SPELLINGS: m, -mb, -lm, -mn

Production *(bilabial nasal resonant)*

The lips close, voice is directed through the open nasopharyngeal port to the nasal cavity and out the nostrils. The tongue lies flat in the mouth or is prepared for the following vowel sound providing opening for resonation of the voice in the entire oral cavity closed off by the lips, as well as resonation in the opened nasal cavity. The teeth are slightly opened.

Internal Feedback Information

TACTILE: Lips touch with closure. Voicing may be felt.

AUDITORY: Voicing may be heard.

Sensory Instructional Possibilities

TACTILE: Vibration of voicing easily felt on the lips, nose, or cheeks. Some emission of breath from nostrils.

VISUAL: Lip closure is easily visible.

Suggestions for Development

1. Imitate from teacher's model; *avoid* producing with lips pressed tightly together.

2. Let the student feel voice vibration on the sides of the nose and on the lips. Vibration may also be felt on top of head.

3. If the student can produce oral resonant vowels but cannot imitate **m**, have him produce -**u**- and extend it. While the vowel is being sounded, have the student close his lips and continue phonating.

Common Errors and Suggestions for Improvement

1. Excessive pressure of lips during production: Contrast formation with excessive pressure to that of appropriate pressure. Have student imitate teacher's production of a series of **mumumumumumumu**- uttered at a slow rate with obvious relaxation of the facial muscles. Have the student produce an extended **m**; flick down his lower lip rapidly to give the idea of relaxing his lips. Place the student's finger between your lips giving different degrees of pressure; indicate pressure which is appropriate for **m** closure.

2. Tongue closure reducing the volume of the oral cavity for resonance: Redevelop the **m** showing student that the tongue lies flat in the mouth. Use a diagram, showing that the tongue does not make closure either at the alveolar ridge, or at the palate or velum. Let the student feel vibration on the lips with correct production of **m**. With tongue closure, lip vibration will be reduced.

*3. Extended duration of **m** in connected speech:* Practice **mumumumumumu**- uttered rapidly on a single breath.

*4. Smacking of lips or insertion of **b** following **m** before a vowel:* Write "b" between **m** and vowel; cross it out to show nature of error. Have student produce syllables with **m** in a very relaxed way. Produce a series of **mumumumu-mumu**- very rapidly. Have the student produce an extended **m**; gently move his jaw downward to open for a vowel. Write a small "h" between the **m** and following vowel to show a relaxation between the sounds as "m__ h ee__."

*5. Substitution of **b** for **m**, an oral for nasal error:* If substitution is caused by excessive pressure of lips on closure, reduce pressure as described in #1 above. Write the letter "b" and cross it out to show the nature of the error. Develop in a syllable **mee**, extending the duration of **m**. Develop in a syllable **eem** with extended duration of **m**.

6. *Non-vocalized breath emitted through nose before or during* **m** *sound:* Practice prolonged humming on a single breath. Demonstrate that there is little noticeable breath emission in appropriate production on back of student's hand; contrast with unacceptable breath emission.

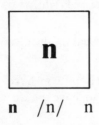

n   /n/   n

KEY WORDS: **n**ew, ti**n**, a**ny**
SPELLINGS: n, kn-, pn-, gn-, -gn

Production *(lingua-alveolar nasal resonant)*

The tip of the tongue closes against the alveolar ridge and the sides of the tongue against molars, the teeth and lips are open, voice is directed through the nasal cavity and out the nostrils. The back of the tongue is open to the oropharynx both for resonation of voice in the oral cavity closed off by the tip of the tongue at the alveolar ridge, and for resonation in the opened nasal cavity. Tongue pressure at the alveolar ridge is less than for the **t** or **d**. The acoustic difference between **m** and **n** depends on the differences in size and shape of the oral cavity, closed at the lips for **m**, and closed by the tongue and alveolar ridge for **n**.

Internal Feedback Information

TACTILE: Tip of the tongue touches the alveolar ridge. Voicing can be felt.

KINESTHETIC: Movement of the tongue slightly upward to the alveolar ridge.

AUDITORY: Voicing may be heard.

Sensory Instructional Possibilities

TACTILE: Vibration of voicing can be easily felt on the nose. Some emission of breath from nostrils can be felt.

VISUAL: Raised tongue point can be seen through the slightly open teeth.

Suggestions for Development

1. Imitate from teacher's model; let student feel voice vibration on the nose.

2. Develop by analogy from **m** for manner of production. Show the student the closure of the point of tongue and alveolar ridge. By diagram show that

the back of the tongue does not close with the velum or palate. Have **m** and **n** repeated in close succession.

3. Develop by analogy from **d** for place of production. Have student take the tongue position for **d** if he has already developed that sound. Let him feel voice vibration on the nose as the tongue position is held.

4. If good tongue closure is not made, **n** can be developed in steps of gradually withdrawing the tongue point. First have the **n** produced with the tongue point protruding slightly between the closed lips; a sound between the **m** and **n** will result. Next have student pull the tongue in just inside the lips to produce the sound. When this is successful, have student open his lips, making the tongue closure with the upper lip. Then make the closure just behind the teeth, and finally on the alveolar ridge.

Common Errors and Suggestions for Improvement

1. Back of the tongue raised to close off the oral cavity; sound produced will be between **ng** *and* **n**: Show student by diagram that the back of the tongue is down leaving the oral cavity open in the back. Redevelop by analogy from **d**, as described above. Have student produce a series of **nu-nu-nu-nu-** syllables with the mouth wide open. When the **n** is produced, have student narrow opening of mouth.

2. Inadequate closure of the tongue and alveolar ridge: Redevelop by analogy from **d** or **t**. Redevelop following steps of #4, above. Demonstrate with mirror that the tongue is spread wide for complete closure.

3. Tongue pressure too great on closure: Practice rapid repetitions of **n** with a vowel as in **nununununu-**, on a single breath. Demonstrate reduced pressure by showing appropriate pressure with teacher's thumb on palm of student's hand.

ng

ng / ŋ / ng

KEY WORDS: so**ng**, si**ng**er
SPELLINGS: -ng, -n(k),
-n(g) (single),
-n(x)

Production *(lingua-velar nasal resonant)*

The back of the tongue closes against front portion of velum or back portion of palate, the teeth and lips are open, voice is directed through the nasal cavity and out the nostrils. The tip of the tongue rests just behind the lower front teeth forming a resonating cavity in the front of the open mouth.

Internal Feedback Information

TACTILE: Closure of back of tongue on velum or palate gives little information; voicing may be felt.

KINESTHETIC: Raising of back of tongue to close against velum or palate gives little information; closure lighter than for **k** or **g**.

AUDITORY: Voicing can be heard.

Sensory Instructional Possibilities

TACTILE: Vibration of voicing with fingers on nose, some nasal emission of air.

VISUAL: Place of production visible only with exaggerated mouth opening.

Suggestions for Development

1. Demonstrate the position of the tongue by opening the mouth wide, then slowly narrowing the opening; produce the **ng**, letting the student feel the voice vibration on the nose.

2. Develop by analogy from **m** and **n** for manner of production. Point out that closure of the mouth moves back from **m** to **n** to **ng**. Use the analogy of **b** to **d** to **g** to show the position of lips and tongue closure for **m**, **n**, and **ng**, respectively.

3. With the mouth slightly open, have student emit breath through the nose; then have student vocalize the breath.

4. Have the student produce **n** while the teacher holds down the tip of his tongue with the tip of her finger or a tongue depressor.

5. With thumb and forefinger on either side of the student's neck below the base of the tongue, press gently upward and hold the position; indicate nasality by touching the side of the nose.

Common Errors and Suggestions for Improvement

1. Closure made too far back on velum and tongue: With diagrams compare correct and incorrect placement. Have student keep front of tongue against lower front teeth while producing **ng**. Practice **ng** in syllables with **ee** and other vowels with forward tongue placement.

*2. Inserting the sounds **k** or **g** after the* **ng:** Demonstrate by tactile impression on the back of the hand that no explosion of breath is present. Redevelop by analogy from **m** and **n**, using syllables such as **mee nee ngee** to show transition from nasal consonant to following vowel. Then produce syllables initiated by a vowel such as **eem een eeng**.

3. Preceding vowel is given nasal resonance: Practice syllables beginning with another consonant blended with the extended vowel and concluded by **ng**: as **weeeeeeng, woooooong**.

4. Following vowel is given nasal resonance: Write a small "g" after the **ng** to show that the tongue/velum contact is discontinued as in "sing g ing."

l /l/ **l**

KEY WORDS: low, bowl, color
SPELLINGS: l, ll, -le, -el

Production *(lingua-alveolar lateral resonant)*

The nasopharyngeal port closes, the tip of the tongue is closed with slight pressure against the alveolar ridge with opening on both sides, voicing escapes on both sides of the tongue between the tongue and molars, and out the oral cavity. The mouth opening is that for the preceding and following vowels. The **l** is voiced when it initiates a syllable and when it is preceded by a voiced consonant (**bl-, gl-,** as in *blue* and *glass*). The **l** is given without voice when it is preceded by a breath consonant (**pl-, kl-, sl-, fl-,** as in *play, clean, slow,* and *fly*), modifying the flow of air from the previous breath consonant. In most consonant blends, the **l** tongue position should be taken before the previous consonant is initiated.

When **l** follows sounds articulated by the tongue in approximately the same place as **l** (examples: **t, d, n**), the tongue tip maintains its position for the preceding sound which is released into the **l** position by opening the sides of the tongue (*bottle, cradle, channel*).

When **l** is the final consonant following another consonant (as in *cable, angle, bottle, gavel*), the **l** becomes a semi-vowel and is produced as a syllable. With the tongue touching the alveolar ridge as described above, the mouth open and lip position are those as for the vowel **-u-**.

Internal Feedback Information

TACTILE: Tip of the tongue touches the alveolar ridge. Voicing can be felt.

KINESTHETIC: Movement of the tongue slightly upward to alveolar ridge.

AUDITORY: Voicing may be heard.

Sensory Instructional Possibilities

TACTILE: Vibration of voicing felt on the cheeks.

VISUAL: Raised tongue point can be seen through the slightly open teeth.

Suggestions for Development

1. Imitate from the teacher's model on syllables **la(r) la(r) la(r) la(r)**; avoid moving the jaw on producing these syllables.

2. Demonstrate the place of production by opening the mouth wide, showing the tongue tip against the alveolar ridge; point out the apertures on both sides, reduce the mouth opening to normal and produce a steady **l**.

3. Demonstrate the position of the tongue by placing its point on the upper lip, point out the apertures on both sides of the tongue, draw it back slowly to position on the alveolar ridge and produce a steady **l**. Let the student imitate, using a mirror if necessary. *Note:* in normal position the tongue tip would be broader than its fine point as it closes against the alveolar ridge.

Common Errors and Suggestions for Improvement

1. Duration too great: Practice production in a quick series of repetitive syllables as **la(r) la(r) la(r) la(r) la(r)**. Produce a series with different vowels in sequence as **la(r) loo lee li-e** on a single breath. Practice in blends with **l** followed by a stop breath consonant as in *help, built, milk.*

*2. Vowel sound -u- between **l** and following vowel:* Have student first take the position for the following vowel and then elevate the tongue for **l**. Produce the blend without dropping the jaw on **loo, lee, law.**

*3. Substitution of **n** for **l**, a nasal/oral error:* Demonstrate the tactile difference by having the student feel vibration on the nose for nasalized **l**. Practice a series of syllables beginning with a vowel as in **a(r)la(r)la(r)la(r)**. Have the student point his tongue outside the mouth; demonstrate that it may be slowly pulled back inside the mouth to touch the alveolar ridge, keeping the tongue pointed and narrow. If necessary, have the child occlude his nostrils making a series of **la(r)** syllables.

4. Tongue raised in back of the mouth for production: Have the student point his tongue outside the mouth, slowly pulling it inside the mouth, keeping it pointed and narrow as it touches the alveolar ridge; reduce mouth opening toward normal and produce a series of **la(r)** syllables. Use a mirror to help student with this exercise.

r

r /r/ r-

KEY WORDS: red, bar, oral
SPELLINGS: r, rr, wr-, -rrh

Production *(lingua-palatal resonant)*

The nasopharyngeal port closes, the tongue tip is turned up toward the palate just behind the alveolar ridge but without touching, the sides of the tongue are against the upper molars, voicing escapes between the tongue and palate and out the oral cavity. Duration is short. The lips are not rounded but may be slightly protruded as with $\overset{2}{oo}$; lips generally take the position of surrounding vowels. The tongue may be curled back—retroflexed.

The **r** is voiced when it initiates a syllable and when it is preceded by a voiced consonant (**br-, dr-, gr-,** as in *brown, dry, grow*). The **r** is given without voice when it is preceded by a breath consonant (**pr-, tr-, kr-, fr-, thr-,** as in *pry, try, cry, fry, three*), modifying the flow of air from the previous breath consonant. In most consonant blends, the **r** tongue position should be taken before the previous consonant is initiated.

In Southern and Eastern U.S. dialects, the **r** following a long vowel (**ee, oo**) or a diphthong is generally replaced with the vowel **-u-**. The final **-er** is also replaced with the vowel **-u-** in words of more than one syllable. In monosyllable words ending in "r," the **r** is dropped but the vowel is slightly prolonged. When **r** is followed by another consonant (*park, bird, surd*), the **r** is dropped but the vowel is slightly prolonged.

Internal Feedback Information

TACTILE: Voicing can be felt.

KINESTHETIC: Movement of the tongue toward the palate can be perceived. If retroflexed, the **r** provides considerable kinesthetic feedback.

AUDITORY: Voicing may be heard.

Sensory Instructional Possibilities

TACTILE: Vibration of voicing felt on cheeks and under chin near base of the tongue.

VISUAL: Elevation of tongue can be seen through the slightly open teeth.

Suggestions for Development

1. Imitate from teacher's model in syllables; demonstrate place of production by opening mouth wide, show the tongue raised but not touching the palate, narrow mouth opening to normal, produce **r** followed by various vowels.

2. Diagram tongue position with the tip slightly turned back. Using one hand to designate the palate and the other the tongue, show that the tongue tip is raised for initial **r** and then lowered for formation of the following vowel.

3. Develop by analogy from **l**. Have the student produce extended **l**, gradually pulling his tongue back. Use diagram to show positions for **l** and for **r**.

4. Develop by analogy from **th** and **z**. Show student that the tongue is pulled back successively for production of **th** to **z** to **r**. *Avoid* letting the student produce **r** with fricative quality resulting from excessive breath flow.

5. Develop breath **r** in association with **p, k, f, t, th** on blends. On **pr-** and **fr-** blends, the tongue position for **r** can be taken before the **p** or **f** is produced. Practice these breath blends first without a vowel following. When they can be produced easily, add a vowel for syllables such as **proo, pra(r), pree**. Contrast syllables **proo/broo, pra(r)/bra(r)**, and **pree/bree**.

6. For the student who cannot raise his tongue adequately for **r** production because of muscular control problems, an alternate formation is to produce **r** with the tongue against the upper molars on one side.

7. Have the student produce **zh**; push the tongue up and back with tongue depressor or pencil eraser while the **zh** continues.

Common Errors and Suggestions for Improvement

1. Substitution of **w** *for* **r**: Redevelop showing that the tongue is raised toward the palate; do not let student protrude and round the lips.

2. Vowel sound **-u-** *inserted between* **r** *and following vowel:* Have student first take the position for the following vowel and then elevate the tongue for **r**. Produce the blend without dropping the jaw on **roo, ree, raw**.

3. Vowel sound **-u-** *inserted between* **r** *and preceding consonants:* Develop **r** as a breath consonant after **p, t, k, th, f**. To blend with **b**, student should take the lip position for **b** (closure) while the tongue is in the **r** position, as in *brown*.

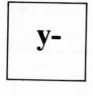

y-   /j/   y

Production *(lingua-palatal resonant glide)*

With voice, the nasopharyngeal port closes, the lips are slightly pulled back; the tip of the tongue remains behind the lower front teeth and the front of the tongue is raised toward the palate. Tongue/palate aperture is slightly smaller and farther back than for **ee**. The **y** is always released into a vowel; taking the tongue and lip formation above, the **y** is very brief, rapidly gliding into the formation of the following vowel.

Internal Feedback Information

TACTILE: Voicing may be felt.

KINESTHETIC: Raising of tongue and pulling back of lips.

AUDITORY: May be heard in a syllable, but duration is short.

Sensory Instructional Possibilities

TACTILE: Vibration of voicing felt by hand on cheeks or under chin.

VISUAL: Slight pulling back of lips.

Suggestions for Development

1. Develop **y** in syllables using a wide variety of vowels; emphasize the relatively short duration of the **y** in relation to the following vowel.

2. Imitate from teacher's model. Show student with mirror that **y** is similar to **ee**, but demonstrate that the duration is shorter.

3. In the syllable **yee**, demonstrate by diagram that the raised tongue is slightly farther back for **y** than for **ee**, and that in the blend of **y** and **ee** the raised tongue moves slightly forward.

Common Errors and Suggestions for Improvement

1. Duration too great (similar to duration of **ee***):* By underlining, show stu-

dent that **y** is shorter than **ee** as follows: "y<u>ee</u>." Write syllables with **y** underlining the vowel and only the last part of the **y** as follows: "y<u>oo</u>."

2. Produced with audible breath friction, heard as **h**: Reduce duration. Demonstrate the lack of breath flow by tactile impression on student's hand.

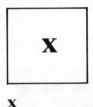

x

KEY WORDS: bo**x**, ta**xi**
SPELLINGS: -x, -ks, -cks

Production *(lingua-velar, lingua-alveolar breath affricate)*

This sound is essentially an affricate combining **k** and **s**. The position for stop
k is taken and released into the **s** position with a single impulse.

Suggestions for Development

Have the student take mouth opening for **s** before producing the **k** portion. If
the **k** and **s** are written, connect the two with a line to show they are one
sound.

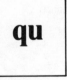

qu

KEY WORDS: **qu**een, li**qu**id
SPELLINGS: qu-

Production *(lingua-velar, bilabial breath affricate)*

This sound is essentially an affricate combining **k** and **wh**. The position for
stop **k** is taken and released into the **wh** position with a single impulse.

Suggestions for Development

Have the student take mouth and lip position for **wh** before producing the **k**
portion. If the "k" and "wh" are written, connect the two with a line to show
they are one sound.

Front Vowels

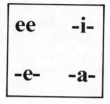

ee / i / e

KEY WORDS: **east, beet, be**
SPELLINGS: -e, ea, -ee, -ey,
         -ie-, (c)ei-

-i- / ɪ / i

KEY WORDS: **if, bit**
SPELLINGS: i-, -y-, -ee-

-e- / ɛ / e

KEY WORDS: **end, bet**
SPELLINGS: e-, -ea-, -ue-,
         -ei-, -e(r)e

-a- / æ / a

KEY WORDS: **at, mat**
SPELLINGS: a-, -au(gh), -ai-

Production

The middle and front portion of the tongue is raised high with the tip of the tongue touching behind the lower front teeth. The sides of the back of the tongue touch the upper molars laterally. The lips are not directly involved but tend to retract at the corners as the front of the tongue is raised. For **ee** the tongue is arched high almost to the palate and the upper and lower front teeth nearly contact each other. For **-i-** the tongue arch is not so high and the opening between the teeth is increased slightly. The tongue height decreases and teeth opening increases further for **-e-** and further still for **-a-**. The lateral contact of the tongue and upper molars may be broken for **-a-**.

Suggestions for Development

Develop in syllables with initial and final consonants. The forward arching of the tongue is essential for the definitive production of these vowels. Emphasize the tongue position with a mirror, first exaggerating the mouth opening for tongue visibility and then closing the mouth opening for production of the vowel. Demonstrate the forward arching of the tongue by projecting the middle of the tongue forward of the teeth while the tip remains behind the lower front teeth; then slowly withdraw the tongue inside the mouth while decreasing the mouth opening and produce the vowel **ee.**

Give a similar demonstration for **-i-, -e-,** and **-a-,** lowering the tongue successively for each of the vowels. Develop **-i-, -e-, -a-** by analogy from **ee.** Using a mirror, imitate a series of **ee, -i-, -e-, -a-,** pointing out the difference in mouth opening. Draw a series of diagrams showing both the lowering of the tongue arching and the increasing mouth opening successively for each of the vowels.

Develop **ee** in association with **h.** If the student can produce **h,** have him do so with the mouth opening for **ee,** adding voice to the breath **h.** Practice a series of **h, h, hee.** To restrict breath flow sufficiently to feel the friction of **h,** the student will tend to raise his tongue toward the palate approximating the position for producing **ee.** Retracting the corners of the mouth will tend to raise the front of the tongue to the appropriate position for **ee.** If necessary, use this device to raise the tongue, but later show the student production of **ee** without lip retraction which can cause tension.

Develop **ee** in association with **sh.** The position for **sh** is similar to the **ee.** Practice in syllables **shee, shee, shee.**

Common Errors and Suggestions for Improvement (See also pages 181-182.)

1. Imprecision (a common error of vowels where production is slightly off target so that **-e-** sounds like **-a-**): show student openings of mouth contrasting one position with another in isolation and in various combinations.

2. Indefiniteness (another common error for vowels, with tongue arching lacking or inadequate so that these vowels sound something like **-u-,** the neutral vowel): Redevelop vowels demonstrating the frontal arching of the tongue. Use a mirror, a model, or diagrams as necessary to show the position of the tongue for these vowels. With the tongue tip behind the lower front teeth, practice with a mirror, arching and protruding the tongue, then returning it inside the mouth still arched toward the palate. Let the student insert his finger into the teacher's mouth to feel proximity of tongue to palate and degree of upward pressure.

3. Rigidity (in attempting to arch the tongue upward, the lower jaw may be held rigidly with teeth clenched and lips drawn back too far): Using a mirror, demonstrate the child's exaggerated tension compared to the appropriate level of relaxation. Conduct tongue exercises taking care to see that there is not excess tension of lips and jaw.

Back Round Vowels

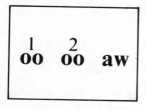

oo̍ /u/ o͞o   KEY WORDS: b**oo**t, t**oo**
                      SPELLINGS: -oo, -ou, -ui, -o,
                                    -oe, -ew, -ough

oo̎ /ʊ/ o͝o   KEY WORDS: b**oo**k, p**u**t
                       SPELLINGS: -o-, -u-, -ou-

aw /ɔ/ ô   KEY WORDS: **aw**ful, c**aug**ht, l**aw**
                       SPELLINGS: au-, aw, a(ll), -o-,
                                    ough(t), -augh(t)

Production

The back of the tongue is raised high with the tip of the tongue touching behind the lower front teeth. The lips are rounded and slightly protruded. For oo̍ the lip aperture is rounder and smaller than for any other vowel, and is almost imperceptibly wider than for **w** (compare in syllable w**oo̍**). For oo̎ the tongue is slightly lower, the jaw is slightly more open, and the lips round but more open. For **aw** the tongue is slightly lower yet, with the jaw and lips slightly more open, and the lips still rounded.

Suggestions for Development

Develop in syllables with initial and final consonants. Emphasize the lip rounding and protrusion which can be seen since this action will tend to raise the back of the tongue. Contrast oo̍ with **a(r)** in series of **a(r)oo̍, a(r)oo̍, a(r)oo̍, a(r)oo̍**; if necessary, have student round his lips around a pencil eraser for oo̍ aperture.

Develop oo̎ by contrast with oo̍. Using a mirror if necessary, imitate a series of oo̍ oo̎ oo̍ oo̎ oo̍ oo̎ oo̍ oo̎ oo̍. Practice oo̎ with initiating and terminating consonants since it generally occurs only between consonants.

Develop **aw** by contrast with oỏ and oỏ. Using a mirror if necessary, imitate a series of oỏ oỏ aw oỏ oỏ aw oỏ oỏ aw. Point out differences in lip opening but continue protrusion and rounding.

Common Errors and Suggestions for Improvement

1. Imprecision and indefiniteness, as in the case of front vowels.

2. Exaggerated or inadequate lip rounding: An exaggerated demonstration for development and the student's quest for tactile-kinesthetic feedback may lead to exaggerated tension on lip rounded vowels. Contrast correct and inappropriate lip tension with a mirror and by having the student feel the teacher's lips.

Mid Back Vowels

```
+-----------+
|           |
|  a(r)     |
|           |
|    -u-    |
|           |
+-----------+
```

a(r) /ɑ/ a(r)

KEY WORDS: odd, father, park
SPELLINGS: o-, a(r), a(l),
             o(rr), ah

Occurs in Northeastern and Southern U.S., and in England as sound for **ar** in **car, farm, bar** without the glide **r.**

-u- /ʌ/ u
     /ə/ ə

KEY WORDS: **up, cup, above,** lemon, cobra
SPELLINGS: u-, o-e, ou, oe, oo (stressed)

Production

The tongue is relaxed and lies low in the mouth with the tip touching behind the lower front teeth and slightly arched at the back of the mouth. The lips are open and unrounded. The **-u-** requires only a small jaw opening with the tongue and lips relaxed. Because of the little effort required, **-u-** is referred to as the natural or the neutral vowel. The **a(r)** is made with the tongue relaxed but the jaws and lips open wider than for any other vowel.

Suggestions for Development

Develop in syllables with initial and final consonants. The **a(r)** is commonly chosen as a first vowel to develop. Develop in a series of syllables **la(r) la(r) la(r) la(r) la(r)**. Develop as a separate vowel, showing student that the tongue lies flat in the mouth. Develop **-u-** by contrast to **a(r)**, demonstrating the reduced mouth opening for **-u-**. Practice **-u-** in syllables with initial and final consonants rather than as an individual sound. When **-u-** is unstressed, its duration should be brief.

Common Errors and Suggestions for Improvement

1. Tongue withdrawn from front teeth and arched high in mouth: This error may be accompanied by nasal emission if tongue arch touches velum or palate. Open the mouth wide, show student that the tongue touches the lower front teeth and lies flat in the mouth; reduce mouth opening and phonate. Have student protrude tongue beyond front teeth, then pull it back, touching back of lower front teeth. If nasal emission is present, have student feel difference in vibration on nose. If necessary, close off student's nostrils to force oral emission.

2. Mouth opening too wide: Relax the jaw and demonstrate reduced opening. Practice in syllables **bu- bu- bu- bu- bu-** and **ba(r) ba(r) ba(r) ba(r) ba(r)** at a fast rate using a mirror to show that the jaw does not drop excessively.

Mixed Vowels

ur /ɝ/   er
    /ɚ/
    /ɜ/

KEY WORDS: **urn, burn, fur**
SPELLINGS: -er, ur, ir, -or-,
ear-, -ar, -re

Production

In the United States the **ur** is made with tongue positions ranging from the / ɜ / to a very strongly retroflexed / ɝ /. Its production and development vary greatly.

General American / ɝ / *stressed,* / ɚ / *unstressed:* See the formation for **r-**. The **ur** is of greater duration than **r-**, carrying full syllable duration (compare *trait/obliterate*). Following consonant **r-**, the **ur** requires movement of the tongue from and again toward the **r-** position (compare *bore/borer*) so that the **ur** approaches a diphthong. Initial **ur** (*irk, urn, urban*) stressed also has diphthong quality as the tongue moves toward the raised position. The **r** coloring may be produced by either raising the tip of the tongue or by holding the central part of the tongue slightly higher than for the vowel / ɜ /.

Southern U.S., Eastern U.S. / ɜ / *stressed:* This is produced without the **r** glide. The tongue lies flat and low in both the front and back. The mouth opening is less than for **-u-** with only a slight opening of the teeth (compare *bud/bird*). The / ɜ / may be combined with / ɔ / on stressed syllables to form a diphthong / ɜɔ /. The unstressed **ur** is very close to the neutral vowel / ə /.

Suggestions for Development

If it is desired to develop the sound with a glide **r**, the / ɝ / should follow development of **r** (see suggestions for development of **r-**). Develop / ɜ / by comparison with **a(r)** and **-u-**, showing the decreasing mouth opening from **a(r)** to **-u-** to **ur**. Demonstrate the narrow separation of the teeth by inserting a flat tongue blade between the teeth, having the student produce **ur** while holding the tongue blade.

Common Errors and Suggestions for Improvement

1. Substitution of **w-** *or* **o͞o** *for* **ur** (/ ɝ /): Redevelop showing that the tongue is raised toward the palate; do not let student protrude and round the lips.

2. Indefiniteness: Develop as with **r-**, demonstrating the tongue tip up toward the palate.

Diphthongs

a-e i-e o-e

ou oi u-e

			Radical	Glide	
a-e	/eɪ/	ā	-i-/-e- /e/	**ee**	KEY WORDS: able, made, may SPELLINGS: ai-, -ay, ei-
i-e	/aɪ/	ī	**a(r)**	**ee/-i-**	KEY WORDS: ice, mice, my, eye SPELLINGS: -i-, i-e, -y, ie, -igh, -ui-
o-e	/ou/	ō	**aw/oo** /o/	$\overset{1}{oo}$	KEY WORDS: old, boat, no, owe SPELLINGS: -o-, o-e, ow, oa-, ough, -ew
ou	/aʊ/	ou	**a(r)**	$\overset{2}{oo}/\overset{1}{oo}$	KEY WORDS: out, now, loud SPELLINGS: ou-, ow, -au-, -ough
oi	/ɔɪ/	oi	**aw**	**ee/-i-**	KEY WORDS: oil, coin, boy SPELLINGS: oi-, -oy

			Glide	Radical	
u-e	/ju/	y͞o͞o	**ee**	$\overset{1}{oo}$	KEY WORDS: use, cute, few, ewe SPELLINGS: u-e, u-, -ue-, -ew, -ou

Production

Diphthongs have two parts, a short portion called a glide or vanish, and a longer portion called a radical or nucleus. The prime characteristic in formation of the diphthong is movement from one part to the other within a single syllable. Diphthongs **a-e, i-e, o-e, ou,** and **oi** feature movement from the radical to the glide, while **u-e** moves from the glide to the radical.

Suggestions for Development

Develop in syllables with initial and final consonants. Develop by imitation as new vowels, emphasizing the movement from radical to glide or glide to radical, and associating the diphthong with its written symbol. If necessary, develop as two simple vowels the student has already learned, emphasizing the continuous movement from one to the other. Demonstrate the connection by joining the two portions with a continuous line as "ee____oo" for **u-e.** If diphthongs are developed as two vowels, we suggest the following simple vowel combinations for diphthongs:

$$a\text{-}e = \text{-}e\text{-} + ee; \; i\text{-}e = a(r) + ee; \; oi = aw + ee;$$
$$o\text{-}e = aw + \acute{o}o; \; ou = a(r) + \acute{o}o; \; u\text{-}e = ee + \acute{o}o.$$

To demonstrate the two positions of a diphthong, draw two sets of parallel lines representing lip openings for the radical and glide; connect the lines to show the continuous movement from one opening to the other as follows:

i-e = a(r) ee

To suggest the difference in duration, make the glide portion shorter than the radical. To suggest the difference in intensity, write the radical portion of the diphthong in strong solid lines and the glide portion in softer dotted lines, or write the radical portion larger than the glide.

Common Errors and Suggestions for Improvement

1. Omission of the glide: Redevelop, emphasizing the two positions of the diphthong. If necessary, exaggerate the duration and intensity of the glide.

2. Prolongation of the glide: Redevelop demonstrating the short duration and reduce intensity of the glide with diagrams as suggested for development. Practice in syllables terminated with stop consonants.

3. Overall duration of diphthong too great: Seeking to achieve the two positions of the diphthong, the student may extend the overall duration beyond that of a typical syllable. Practice diphthongs in a series of syllables with simple vowels such as **boot, boot, bote, bawt,** having student keep equal duration on each of the syllables. The teacher may use a metronome or have the student move his arm in cadence to attempt equal duration.

CHAPTER V

Developing Speech

In this chapter we shall be concerned with the child who when first encountered has little or no speech, and with the teacher's role in developing his speech. Given the encouraging trend toward early identification and assessment of hearing impaired children, the need for teacher involvement of whatever degree or kind is likely to be recognized sometime below the age of 5 and in most instances much sooner.

METHODS FOR DEVELOPING SPEECH

In selecting a "method" or what may be called a general strategy, we recommend that the teacher have access to an array of alternatives whose applicability to developing speech has been demonstrated by experience. In this section we shall delineate what we consider to be three prominent alternative methods. Of course, there are accommodating variations subsumed under each method and there are overlapping or common elements, but as a general proposition the methods are discrete and distinctive enough to merit separate treatment. In a sense, they constitute a gradient of instructional requirements concentrating primarily on the degree of teacher control and direction involving the unit of speech input to and production by the child, the extent of purposeful drilling, and the relative emphasis on particular sensory channels or combinations of them to transmit information about speech and its feedback. We have puzzled over how to label these methods. For convenience of

147

communication, we shall label them the "Auditory Global," "Multisensory Syllable Unit" and "Association Phoneme Unit" methods. What is important is not the labels but the exposition of the methods which in turn give significance to the labels.

Auditory Global Method

The principal features of the Auditory Global method are that the primary, although not always exclusive, channel for speech development is auditory and that the input is fluent connected speech. The terms "Auditory-Oral," "Aural-Oral," "Acoupedic," "Natural," and "Unisensory" (auditory) are conventionally used as synonyms for the same fundamental method or to designate variations within the same general framework (7, 32, 53, 64, 73). The essential characteristics of the method are: (1) maximum emphasis on use of hearing, (2) comprehensive intervention, well beyond the traditional school setting, and (3) emphasis on connected speech.

1. Maximum Emphasis on Use of Hearing

The undergirding premise, elaborated in Chapter III, of the Auditory Global method is that the most useful way to achieve intelligible speech is input of spoken language to the child's auditory channel, however much its sensitivity is reduced. The more enthusiastic among its advocates say, "There is no such thing as a totally deaf child," and, "Every remnant of hearing is usable for developing oral communication." Even if one disagrees with this rather extreme position, the data mentioned in the Introduction on the hearing status of children in schools for deaf children reported by the Center for Demographic Studies at Gallaudet College do point to a substantial number of children with hearing that, if cultivated, would facilitate the development of their speech. Such cultivation, if it is to be productive, demands of the teacher (or whoever is responsible for management of the child) that she ensure that the following key requirements are met:

a. Early use of amplification: Amplification should begin as soon as the child's hearing loss has been identified and need not wait for absolute determination of the nature and degree of hearing loss. Even before definitive selection of a hearing aid is made, everyday situations in an infant's life can be exploited to accomplish amplification, such as speaking close to the child's ear and raising the voice without shouting. There is disagreement among audiologists as to the earliest age when it is advisable to recommend that a hearing aid be worn. Some would advise a hearing aid immediately upon identification of hearing loss, however young the child may be. The more conservative view is to establish some confidence about the degree and nature of

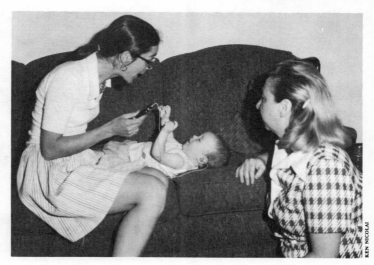

Baby's first hearing aid. Guiding parent in its use.

a child's loss. Nevertheless, proponents of the Auditory Global method generally would prefer that by the age of 6 months, given identification, a hearing aid should be advised. As far as we know there are no incontrovertible data on this point. Perhaps the best that can be said is that the ***child-instrument experience***, that is, how the child responds to the instrument, be subject to continuous, careful cognizance, analysis, and guidance by the person responsible for the child's speech development.

b. Periodic re-examination of hearing: The results of the first hearing test, however competently administered, are not often conclusive; nor, as we have pointed out, do they yield much significant information about the hearing of a very young child. Hearing examinations need to be given *regularly* but less frequently as the child grows older and confidence in test results increases. Nevertheless, the staff should be alert to the possibility that hearing can change, and any such suspicion should require audiologic evaluation along with otologic check for an acquired conductive component.

c. Selection of optimum amplification systems: In Chapter III, Ling has described the fundamentally important electroacoustic characteristics of hearing aids as related to speech perception, with emphasis on gain and frequency range. Other requirements for optimum amplification are:

(1) CONSISTENCY OF RESPONSE: If two types of amplification equipment are used (such as a group amplifier and a wearable hearing aid), their frequency response should be fairly similar. Otherwise the child may be hearing speech in one way over one amplifier and quite another way over the other, leading to some confusion in interpreting what he hears.

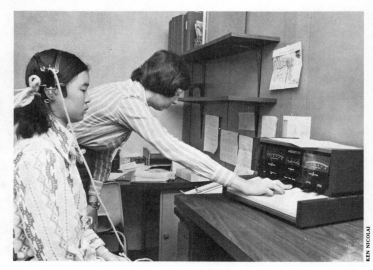

Checking middle ear function using impedance bridge.

(2) SPEAKER FEEDBACK: The hearing aid should amplify the child's own speech.

(3) SOUND LOCALIZATION: Normally-hearing persons tend to turn their heads to sources of sound. Wherever possible, amplification should facilitate this for the hearing impaired child so that he can conveniently search for, locate, and attend to sound. Ideal for this are head-mounted binaural instruments, but for many children—particularly those with severe losses—compromises need to be made.

(4) FREEDOM OF MOVEMENT: The amplification system should provide the greatest possible freedom for the child to move around.

(5) WEARABILITY: The hearing aid should be comfortable to wear, including ear inserts, earphones, and equipment on the body or head. Its maximum power output should be tolerable. This level may be raised with continued usage (194).

(6) SIMPLICITY OF OPERATION: The instrument should not require complicated adjustments and adaptations for teacher and child use whether in setting of controls or in constant handling of microphones. Entangling wires are a hazard and an enticing lure for unnecessary child manipulation, suggesting a sort of "signal to nuisance" ratio.

(7) RUGGEDNESS: This refers to the resistance of an instrument to damage from the inevitable rough handling by children. This is difficult to determine by inspection, but careful sample record keeping of "down time" of particular instruments could furnish useful cues to ruggedness. Perhaps producers

will conduct "shake tests" and repeated manipulation of cords and inserts so that ruggedness can be specified and documented.

d. Periodic examination of the hearing aid: We underline Ling's suggestion that there should be a routine *daily* screening examination of the child's hearing aid by the parents and later by the teacher. This can be done by visual inspection, by battery charge testing, and by listening to sound through the instrument. To permit effective listening, the parent or teacher should have a personal ear mold. A second level of hearing aid examination is through electronic analysis. Hearing aids can and should be analyzed regularly for their electroacoustic characteristics which change with usage and over time (112). Some audiology clinics, schools, and hearing aid distributors have analyzing equipment available.

e. Constant usage of amplification: Finally, we repeat for emphasis the need to ensure constancy of usage and a satisfactory acoustic environment discussed in Chapter II.

2. Comprehensive Intervention

Although systematic and coordinated auditory stimulation is the central focus of the Auditory Global method, it achieves its full potential only if the intervention is timely, broad, comprehensive, and generally individualized. For this method—appreciably more than for other methods—the "classroom" is the child's total environment. He is "in school" all of his waking hours. On the gradient of instructional requirements, teacher control and direction stress at all times the opportunities for acquisition of speech by abundant auditory experience. This is particularly true in the case of the very young child. This is not to say that other methods exclude this need, but rather that in the Auditory Global method it places a greater demand on the teacher's time and energy and occupies a more prominent place in her planning.

At the core of comprehensive intervention is the development and maintenance of a milieu positively responsive to the child's speech output. Even though a child may get some enjoyment from the feedback of his own voice, he is likely to cease talking if he is not encouraged. Responsiveness is especially important to the child with hearing impairment because reduced or absent feedback limits the appreciation of his own voice. Responses may include "primitive" rewards, fulfillment of the purpose of the speech utterance, and related spoken language. Utterances by the very young child should elicit immediate personal-human rewards of smiling, approving words, or affectionate patting. A parent may also invent his own system of auditory-visual rewards such as clapping the hands in response to speech or speech-like sounds. As the child grows older, more tangible rewards such as special privi-

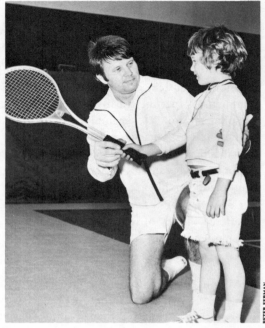

Experiences build language.

PETER FERMAN

leges or items of appealing value may be effective. Such rewards are extrinsic to speech itself and should not be emphasized or continued for long periods. The quality of the utterance and the stage of development of the child's speech should influence reward-giving. This is a matter of judgment. The ultimate reward, of course, should be the satisfaction of having communicated by spoken language. Another kind of rewarding response is directly related to the utterance and should teach a child that speech is generally purposeful. When he says, "want cookie," and receives a cookie, he learns that speech is not only reward-giving but also accomplishes a specific purpose.

A third kind of especially valuable response is the spoken language of the person to whom the child's speech is directed. For the very young child this may be the simple repetition of the speech-like sounds of his babbling and other vocalization. Parents will naturally select for repetition the speech sounds of their native language, thus reinforcing the sounds appropriate to the desired speech pattern. When utterances of the baby resemble words of the language, parents can repeat the words as they usually pronounce them, or perhaps emphasize some aspect of the words—such as accent—so that the child might focus on what he previously may not have perceived. In order that the child begin to use these utterances to communicate, it is important for the parent to indicate the meaning of words to the child by pointing, gesturing, or other means.

3. Emphasis on Connected Speech

A prominent feature of the Auditory Global method is the emphasis on connected speech, whether in response to a child's utterance or initiated—as it frequently should be—by the teacher. Connected speech input to the child is not left to chance. The best acoustic amplification and comprehensive intervention may be ineffective unless the ***amount, nature,*** and ***direction*** of stimuli are taken into account.

a. Amount of connected speech: Increased speech input to the child should begin at a very early age, even though there is no apparent sign from the child that he is understanding what is said. The child with normal hearing is talked to with meaningful connected speech for many months before he produces such signs, and for a year or more before he begins to use even single words. From the time the hearing impaired child wears his first hearing aid and the intervention program begins, parents and teachers must expect to put in a great deal of speech before they can anticipate encouraging responses from the child.

The overall amount of connected speech input should be increased over that which would normally be available to a child without impaired hearing. He should, of course, be exposed to the "small talk" and courtesy phrases which we use daily. With a good amplification system, television offers a valuable source of meaningful speech input. Although lipreading is not easy from the typical television production and not available at all on cartoons, environmental sounds and speech associated with action are available constantly. It is a supplement to live speech input but cannot replace it.

If it can be arranged, the hearing impaired child should have language and speech input from non-impaired children his own age. Such children provide speech models from vocal tracts of the same size. Vowel formant positions will thus be easier to imitate than those of adults. Using connected language, parents and teachers can learn to ***describe*** and ***explain*** what they and the child are seeing or doing. They can ***narrate*** stories and they can ***recapitulate*** experiences. Situations should be arranged to stimulate the child to associate spoken language with observation and action.

b. Nature of connected speech: We caution on two popular oversimplifications about stimulation with connected speech. One is that the parents, teachers, and all people in the child's environment should treat the child exactly as they would a child without hearing loss, talking to him as though he were hearing and understanding all that is said. Another is that these people should "talk, talk, talk" to the child. While such advice stresses the importance of increasing the amount of speech in the child's environment, it frequently neglects the need for tailoring the nature of the connected speech or directing it to the child to compensate for his hearing loss.

The Auditory Global method exploits the strong possibility of attainment by the child of natural **speech rhythm** and **language** competence that contribute invaluably to speech intelligibility. Connected spoken language which is characterized by natural rhythm gives the child the opportunity to hear a model of the important patterns of speech and to imitate them. It is not out of order to conjecture here that the naturally patterned speech of the teacher is likely to be adversely affected, as will the intelligibility of the child's speech, if it must accommodate to the temporal features of simultaneously presented manual signals, especially for very young children. The naturally recurring patterns associated with declarative sentences, questions, and exclamations may be slightly exaggerated in the speech of the teacher to create a flow which the child may imitate in his own speech, even if, as we have seen in Chapter III, his residual hearing is concentrated only in the low frequencies.

By hearing repeated examples of connected speech, the child with normal hearing not only imitates what he hears but formulates inductively what he believes are the rules of spoken language. However, the restricted auditory sensitivity of the hearing impaired child reduces the redundancy and linguistic cues of the language available to him. Nevertheless, there may still be sufficient phonologic, syntactic, and semantic cues to facilitate inductive acquisition of the rules of speech and language. Of course, the connected speech of the teacher should take into account the state of the child's language development as suggested by Simmons-Martin in Figure 18.

When the child has begun to use connected words meaningfully, the parents and teacher can employ the strategy of **expansion** (212). In expanding what the child has said, the adult imitates the child's words, usually retaining the same word order, but adds something to them to form a complete and grammatically correct sentence. For example, if the child has said, "Dog bark," the adult might expand his utterance by saying, "Yes, the dog is barking." This kind of expansion provides the child with a corrective model which informs him that the adult has understood him and is interested. The adult may expect the hearing impaired child to imitate the expanded model at a level appropriate to his stage of development.

After the child has learned to use a number of meaningful words and phrases, the parents and teacher can also use the strategy of **modeling** (213). To model speech and language is to comment relevantly on what the child has said, rather than to improve on it by expansion. If the child has said, "Dog bark," the modeler might say, "Yes, there is a cat in the tree." This not only serves to reward the child but may also enrich his vocabulary and elaborate his syntax.

SKILLS
Reading, writing,
spelling and composing

MATURE LANGUAGE
Involved syntax and reflection
vocabulary of 5000+

CONNECTED LANGUAGE
Simple structure — requests and
questions

LARGER EXPRESSIVE UNITS
Prepositional phrase
Participial phrase

LIMITED EXPRESSIVE LANGUAGE
Naming — Adjectives
Few verbs

IMITATIONS
Actions including mouthing
Sounds including speech

FREE COMPREHENSION
Concepts
Connected language

SITUATIONAL COMPREHENSION
Concrete items
Visible actions

AWARENESS
Concepts
Vocabulary

EXPOSURE

Figure 18. Some steps of language development. Courtesy of A. A. Simmons-Martin, Central Institute for the Deaf.

When the child is very young, the teacher does not attempt deliberately to correct speech sounds, nor does she call specific attention to an error or to poor production of a pattern. Perceived error should guide the classroom activities to help the child move closer to the desired production by increasing in the teacher's own speech the frequency of the indicated model.

c. Directing connected speech to the child: The Auditory Global method stresses the auditory signal as primary speech information supplemented by visual, "real" speech information. Throughout we have repeated the importance of proper use of sound amplification. For example, proper microphone technique is important. To avoid "pattern distortion" the microphone should be held a little to the side of the teacher's mouth so that her direct breath stream will not cause plosives and fricatives to be heard as extra syllables. However, holding the microphone too far from hers or the child's mouth may cause the speech signal to fall below classroom noise levels, and moving a microphone too quickly or not quickly enough may cause failure of parts of the signal to be transmitted over the acoustic amplifier. In addition, we believe speech development can be aided by watching the speaker's face while listening, but that watching all the time is neither necessary nor desirable. Some advocates of versions of the Auditory Global method take pains to see that the child does not receive visual speech information while listening. This persistent "unisensory" emphasis rests on the view that the child should learn to depend on the auditory signal alone in order to develop the fullest use of his hearing. Whether this technique is essential for the development of speech through hearing is still an open question.

To this point our exposition of the Auditory Global method has focused on very young children. This has been intentional since, as we shall see later in this chapter, we shall recommend it for all children as the initial method of choice. However, as the child grows older and we have had sufficient opportunity to observe his progress, specific needs will be revealed that require deliberate attention. The child's performance may indicate a change to the Multisensory Syllable Unit method or the Association Phoneme Unit method, to be described later, or to a continuation within the framework of what can still properly be labeled the Auditory Global method. Later in this chapter we shall suggest criteria for choice of continuation or switch of method, but here we shall consider important aspects of the continuation of the Auditory Global method. In discussions with teachers of whatever methodological persuasions, we have found some difference of opinion regarding the most suitable procedures for speech development of the child at this stage.

Experience with the Auditory Global method has generally been confined to its use with children of preschool age and younger. As children have "graduated" from it, the choice for their continued speech development (and improvement, correction, and maintenance) has been some form of "integration" with minimal attention to speech, or a "traditional" method like the Multisensory Syllable Unit method. The difficulty seems to stem primarily from the assumption that these are the only choices and secondarily from the question of when and how to make these choices. Although there has not been too much experience with the Auditory Global method at the primary

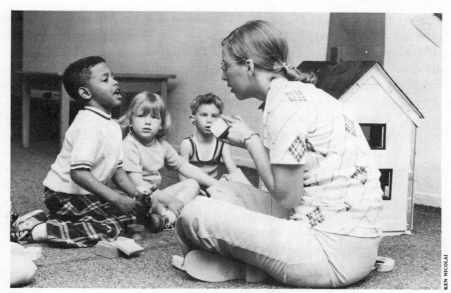

Responding to connected speech input.

and elementary levels, we believe the Auditory Global method is a distinctively viable option beyond the preschool.

It may be properly argued that what we propose as being distinctive about the Auditory Global method beyond preschool should be subsumed under improvement, correction, and maintenance, as discussed in Chapter VI, rather than development. Nevertheless, we believe that some development would still be in process and that no useful, practical purpose is served in trying to establish a fine, indisputable line of demarcation. Our experience leads to a number of pragmatic points about the Auditory Global method as it is continued.

Although the age at which structured and targeted *auditory training* should commence is variable, its usefulness for individual children should be kept in mind. As Ling has reminded us, firm documentation is lacking for the value of particular exercises. However, he does suggest some specific bases for training which we repeat here: discrimination between presence or absence of sound and between loud-quiet, high-low, long-short, sudden-gradual, simple-complex, and steady-changing; ability to use information given by rhythm, stress, intonation, number and rate of syllables; capacity to code, retain, and recall the sequential order of phonemes, words, and sentences spoken; and ability to supply information relative to inaudible items in a sequence on the basis of a knowledge of language that is acquired through previous adaptive experience.

We have noted that *precision of articulation* is the chief need of children whose evaluation suggests continuation by the Auditory Global method. These children are likely to have developed satisfactory patterning and voice quality by the maximum use of hearing, comprehensive intervention, and the emphasis on connected speech. As we shall see when we deal with choices among methods, development of these features of speech is a crucial criterion. Of course, previous procedures need to be continued, but articulation— without sacrifice of achieved fluency—demands more concentrated attention.

At this stage *selective reinforcement* of speech is important. Until now the child has been rewarded for *any* and *all* speech utterances. Unintelligible expression, generally characterized by poor articulation, should not be accepted if it is known that the child has the skill to be intelligible. Helpful here is agreement by parents and teachers on the child's speech capabilities that will influence their expectancies and demands. Practice of selective reinforcement, based on intelligibility, needs to take into account that a child's speech is undoubtedly more intelligible to his teacher and parents than to others. He has given them auditory training. Therefore, what is demanded may require judgment of the probability of whether an utterance would have been understood by listeners not too familiar with the child's speech. This is a subtle judgment that depends on the teacher's confidence in prediction and on the child's skills and attitudes. The teacher will need to seize and, if necessary, contrive opportunities to observe the child speaking to others. This experience should enhance her competence to predict. Where there is no oral atmosphere, these opportunities are unfortunately limited or absent. We simply call attention to this point. Incidentally, it needs to be addressed regardless of the method that is being employed (202).

Mastery of articulation is abetted by equipping the child with a suitable *orthographic system* of the kind described in Chapter I. We recall that we recommend the Northampton symbols with gradual progression to diacritical markings used in standard dictionaries. The child now learns to sound out words. Written symbols are generally associated with sounds in words rather than in isolation. Nevertheless, situations may call for attention to a sound in isolation, but a child should not be considered to "have" a sound until it is given correctly in the variety of phonetic and linguistic contexts in which it occurs in spoken language. This provides the child with the power of attack on the pronunciation of new words and gives the teacher a visual code of communication about speech that is used by his culture. The language of other aspects of speech production can now be introduced to facilitate communication about it. Important among these are structure and function of the speech mechanism and their related vocabulary having to do with manner and place of production—such as breath (voiceless), voice, plosive, fricative, palate, ve-

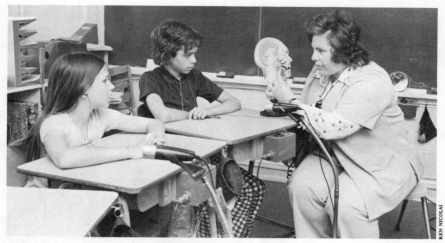

Explaining speech terms.

lum—and descriptive adjectives such as soft, loud, high and low. Diagrams, mirror demonstrations, and films are helpful.

Multisensory Syllable Unit Method

The Multisensory Syllable Unit method is popularly considered to be the "traditional" method of teaching speech to the hearing impaired. We hasten to point out that we do not use the term *traditional* in any pejorative sense. On the contrary, its value has been historically demonstrated by the substantial number of those who have achieved impressive functional speech. Of course, the Multisensory Syllable Unit method has much in common with the Auditory Global method, but its more distinctive characteristics are: (1) multisensory stimulation for speech, (2) focus on the development of speech sounds, and (3) the syllable as the basic unit for speech instruction.

1. Multisensory Stimulation for Speech

The visual, tactile, kinesthetic, and auditory senses are used selectively and discriminatingly for speech development. As we have seen in Chapters III and IV, speech sounds vary in their potential for transmission, perception, and feedback over the different sensory systems. Unlike the emphasis in the Auditory Global method, the auditory system, although used as it contributes particularly to patterning and voice quality—is not likely to make a major contribution to the development of articulation. The teacher makes use of the prominent "sensory" features of sounds and their combinations in developing articulation. For example, in the case of the bilabial consonants **p, b,** and **m,** visual information through lipreading and mirror observation can help the child develop each of them. Yet they cannot be discriminated from each other by vision alone or by hearing. The alert teacher exploits perceivable tactile differences in their production by having the child feel the puff of air on the back of his hand from the **p,** comparing the breath **p** to the vibration of voice on **b,** and feeling with his fingertips on the nose for **m** where vibration of voice peaks. Although feedback is accomplished for each of these sounds by the tactile sensation of the lips touching, the teacher may, through demonstration, emphasize the special kinesthetic feedback of **p** caused by relatively greater muscle tension necessary for this breath plosive, and the intense vibro-tactile feedback of **m.**

Tactile feedback.

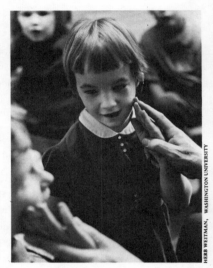

2. Focus on the Development of Speech Sounds

This method assumes that speech will *not* develop just from the child's hearing and seeing connected speech in the course of conversation, however natural or planned. The production of individual sounds, their combination, and speech rhythm need to be learned by focused instruction. Now speech sounds will be introduced a few at a time and in a predetermined order, unlike with the Auditory Global method in which all speech sounds are in some discernible stage of development. A limited number of new sounds may be introduced while other sounds are still in the process of development and still others have already been mastered. The rate and sequence with which new sounds are introduced are governed by the child's progress toward mastery of the sound in combinations.

The order in which speech sounds are developed is important in building up previous experience. Some teachers recommend the same order of development that occurs for children with normal hearing, but others suggest that the limitations of impaired hearing contraindicate this sequence. For them, a useful guide has been to order development based on the ease with which children have been observed to learn the production of sounds. Those sounds which are easiest to learn would be taught first, progressing to sounds of increasing difficulty. The child thus has maximum opportunity for successful experience with speech development. Table 11 shows a consensus of judgments of a sample of teachers experienced in the Multisensory Syllable Unit method about the relative difficulty of developing phonemes. Certainly there are individual differences in judgment. It is interesting, nevertheless, that our *ad hoc* sampling and the data on difficulty of development reported by Hudgins and Numbers agree impressively well (42). Of course, spontaneously produced speech sounds should be reinforced regardless of the order in which they occur. If a child has special difficulty with one sound, the teacher should move on to another rather than persisting.

It is interesting to note here, as we do in our discussion of errors of articulation in Chapter VI, that inadequate coordination of voicing and articulation results in **p** being heard as **b,** **t** as **d,** and **k** as **g** when combined with a vowel. Yet these confusions seldom if ever occur in the production of the isolated consonant. The voice onset time, defined as the interval between the release of the stop closure and the onset of the following vowel, is different for **p** and **b.** It is much shorter for **b,** and if voice onset time is not long enough for **p** it will be heard as **b.** This observation suggests that order of development could take into account classes of combinations that have common features. For example, voiced stops joining vowels (**bu-, du-, gu-**) might be first, then unvoiced stops plus vowels (**pu-, tu-, ku-**). We recall, too, that in Chapter III Ling sug-

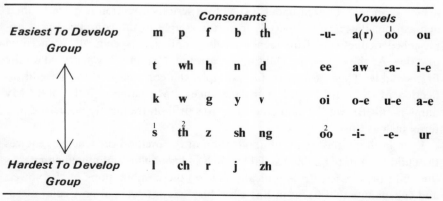

	Consonants					Vowels			
Easiest To Develop Group	m	p	f	b	th	-u-	a(r)	oo	ou
	t	wh	h	n	d	ee	aw	-a-	i-e
	k	w	g	y	v	oi	o-e	u-e	a-e
	s	th	z	sh	ng	oo	-i-	-e-	ur
Hardest To Develop Group	l	ch	r	j	zh				

Table 11. *Rank ordering of groups of phonemes by ease of development, made by teachers of deaf children.*

gests auditory criteria for order of development of sounds. Since no particular order of development has been convincingly validated, it is essential to be alert to all possibilities and to depend on what seems to "work."

Given the Multisensory Syllable Unit method as the general method of choice (as determined by criteria discussed later in this chapter), it is implicit that a period of the day will be set aside for speech work. This period will be devoted to work on development, with introduction at the outset of an orthographic system, as well as to the child's specific needs. The child for whom the Multisensory Syllable Unit method is indicated is likely to require a good deal of repetitive practice and directed drill. It goes without saying that the teacher will be alert to promote transfer of skills acquired in the special period to use in all other situations. As the crucial monitor of the child's speech, she will probably practice more frequent spontaneous correction. Of course, she will exercise discriminating judgment as to what is accepted without correction. Her understanding of a child's capability and motivations will necessarily guide her reinforcing behavior.

3. The Syllable as the Basic Unit for Speech Instruction

This method assumes that extensive use of units smaller than the longer sequences of connected speech is fundamental to instruction. The syllable, as described in Chapter I, is sufficient for coarticulation of phonemes and yet is small enough to allow for accuracy of articulation by not placing too great a demand on motor memory. Furthermore, it is the irreducible unit of speech in which voice quality, inflection, and stress can be demonstrated. The familiar instruction that the "accent is on the __ syllable" illustrates the point.

If the patterns of connected speech are well along, these are, of course, conserved and improved. But where the patterns are arhythmic or nonexistent, articulation may be well under way before serious attention is given to their acquisition. Patterning proceeds from the simple to the complex and is approached deductively from general rules applied to specifically structured practice. At the outset the child may learn that "mother" is accented on the first syllable. Then he learns, for example, the contrast in duration and inflection of the word "Bill" in the sentences, "My name is Bill," and "My name is Bill Brown." The method requires drill on frequently occurring patterns such as this.

Even in the initial stages of application of the method the teacher requires the child to imitate babbled syllables such as **bubububu-** and **mumumumu-**. As the child progresses, drills typically involve the combinations of the vowels and consonants that occur in English. This does not rule out particular attention to single sounds in isolation, but such sounds are not to be considered "learned" until they are produced in conventional syllables.

Since the syllable is the recommended unit of speech, drills should generally be in a syllabic pattern and proceed as the child gains in skills from simple CVC patterns to more complex ones. The order could be CVC (*tot*), CCVC (*stop*), CCCVC (*street*), CVCCC (*desks*). Even within a pattern, varying combinations should be appropriately employed. For example, if the **t** is the phoneme being drilled on, then CVC could include the following patterns, each representing a class of drill:

tVt—vowel changed, initial and final **t** included.

tVp—place changed in final consonant.

pVt—place changed in initial consonant.

tVd—same place but final voicing.

dVt—same place but initial voicing.

tVn—same place but final nasal.

tVs—place and manner changed in final consonant.

If the aim is to drill on plosives preceded by a fricative like ś, then CCVC could be: *stool, spool, skool,* etc. These combinations can also be used for assessment of articulatory skills. Rockey (68), in her phonetic lexicon, has provided an excellent source of monosyllabic and some disyllabic words arranged according to their phonetic structure.

The Association Phoneme Unit Method

The Association Phoneme Unit method was motivated by the need to devise an alternative for those children who by the methods previously described were not learning to talk. It has its origins in the ideas and experience of Mildred McGinnis at Central Institute for the Deaf and was intended for those whose hearing impairment was overlaid by conditions that would render conventional procedures unsuitable to the achievement of oral communication. A number of these conditions and the variety of symptoms ascribed to them were subsumed under the rubric "congenital aphasia." The issues related to etiology, nomenclature, and classification, or whether this clinical entity occurs at all, are beyond the scope of this book, as are any applications of the method to other "learning disabilities." What is pertinent to our purposes is that in our experience hearing impaired children have acquired functional spoken language by this method or its adaptations. This qualifies it for inclusion in our catalogue of methods. Our brief exposition is based on McGinnis' elaboration of the method in her treatise on the identification and education of aphasic children (57) and on our own observation and experience.

The more distinctive characteristics of the Association Phoneme Unit method are these: (1) speech production is associated with other language modalities, (2) the phoneme is the basic unit for speech instruction, and (3) speech development progresses in small increments.

1. Speech Production Is Associated with Other Language Modalities.

The Association Phoneme Unit method is based on the idea that speech perception is influenced by speech production. We tend to hear the speech of others as we produce it. For example, when we hear the Spanish bilabial voiced fricative consonant in *Havana* (a sound that does not occur in English), we hear it either as a **b** (which is a bilabial stop) or a **v** (which is a labio-dental fricative), both sounds which we produce.

The child is taught to produce each sound very precisely, thus developing a strong motor pattern which should be easy for him to remember. He learns to associate most of the speech he sees and hears with the patterns he has produced. No formal lipreading, listening, or reading is attempted in the Association Phoneme Unit method except for words which the child can say.

When a child produces a sound correctly, it is immediately associated with other means of language expression and reception by the following specified steps, generally in the indicated sequence:

a. The child reads the symbol (Northampton) for the sound written by the teacher and pronounces it aloud.

b. He lipreads (and hears as he is able) the sound produced by the teacher and again pronounces it aloud.

c. He lipreads the sound produced by the teacher, writes the appropriate symbol himself, and once more pronounces it aloud.

d. He hears the speech sound—but does not "see" it—as the teacher says it near his ear, then writes it and again pronounces it aloud.

Writing is always associated with oral production. This association of speech with other language modalities is prescribed for a phonologic and linguistic range of increasing complexity from single phonemes, through individual words, to sentences and questions.

2. The Phoneme Is the Basic Unit for Speech Instruction.

The single phoneme in isolation is the basic unit of instruction for speech production. Its precise articulation enhances the memory for the motor acts associated with it and its combinations. Breath sounds (such as **p, f, ch**) are said in isolation without a voice carrier and voiced plosives are terminated with the vowel **-u-**. Since the written symbol is always associated with the spoken phoneme, the child and teacher develop a written inventory of the phonemes which have been "mastered." Near-perfect production of a number of consonants and vowels is required before "blending" of two or more phonemes is attempted. Drills blend consonant and vowel sounds leading to

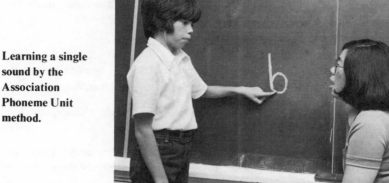

Learning a single sound by the Association Phoneme Unit method.

the articulation of a word. Even after words are begun, the child continues to say the phoneme separately and blended in syllables. When he makes an error in a word, the child is instructed first to repeat the phonemes individually and then to "smooth" the sounds together. To direct attention to individual speech sounds within syllables, consonants are frequently written in one color and the vowels in another. Smoothing may be facilitated by cursive script. Advocates of cursive script point to its clarity in separating words while connecting letters within words.

3. Speech Development Progresses in Small Increments.

From mastery of his first phoneme the child develops speech in small units progressing from the simple to the complex. A reasonable number of individual phonemes are developed before blending of consonants and vowels is attempted. When the child can blend with some confidence, two or more phonemes are combined into single-syllable words such as *pie* and *boat.* When a number of words are mastered, the child is ready to put a few together into simple sentences such as, "I see a boat."

Once the child has learned to recognize and produce a unit of spoken language, he is expected to recall and produce it without frequent prompting. When, for example, the child is asked to say aloud the phoneme associated with a written symbol, the teacher withholds clues until the child has exerted his best effort to respond correctly. The teacher encourages the child to remember and gives him sufficient time to "search his memory." This sort of practice in recall should gradually decrease the time and effort necessary to accomplish it.

For the child who has experienced failure and discouragement by other methods, the experience of success is especially to be stressed. The achievement of real success and its accompanying satisfactions are more probable when the required increment of learning is small.

CHOOSING A METHOD

Recognizing the conditions affecting the acquisition of spoken language, the initial method of choice should meet the following requirements:

1. The method should be appropriate for very young children whenever they are identified.

We enthusiastically advocate appropriately planned measures to develop speech at the earliest possible time. Intervention for speech development could begin at birth. Unfortunately, the opportunity to do this is rare. Such procedures as are available for neonatal screening for hearing impairment are of questionable reliability, validity, and economy, and those that do show some promise are not widely used. Nor is screening routine in "well-baby" clinics or in conventional pediatric care. Even when hearing loss is recognized early, timely intervention does not always follow. Early education programs may not be conveniently available or parents may delay action. Some health care professionals still advise parents to "come back in six months" for more tests or to "wait until he is old enough" for school.

Organized as we now are, our imperfect system of early identification and delays in initiation of action result in the opportunity for intervention coming at different ages for children. In the past, apparent consistency in the age of intervention with deaf children was achieved by setting an arbitrary "age of admission" for enrollment in programs of early education. Such a policy cost children valuable months and even years of waiting until they reached the designated age.

2. The method should provide maximum opportunity for each child to develop his hearing ability, regardless of early estimates of the nature and degree of hearing loss.

Current procedures for assessing and describing the hearing ability of very young children do not yield the information related to speech development that we should like to have. Information about perception of patterns, the use of minimal auditory cues, attentiveness to sound, and sensitivity to changes in intensity, frequency, and duration would be helpful. The younger the child and the greater his hearing impairment, the less information about his hearing ability we can obtain. Many of our audiologic tests require complex directions and responses, previous experience with listening, and, to some extent, familiarity with speech. Firm decisions on the basis of premature and meager evidence should be scrupulously avoided.

Even when reasonably valid audiologic test results (primarily audiograms) are available, audiologists and educators have struggled over the problems of definition and classification for educational purposes. In the main they have resorted to "behavioral" definitions. In this context a *deaf child* is defined as one who "cannot understand and acquire speech and language through the sense of hearing, even with sound amplification," while the *severely hard of hearing child* "suffers delayed speech and language development" (102). But such behavioral definitions are of little value for the young child who, fortuitously, has been identified at an early age. Before these definitions can be applied they require that the child has had some significant experience—has tried and either failed or succeeded. They may also lead to static classification of hearing impaired children into rigidly determined groups in response to traditional arrangements for educational placement.

3. The method should provide an opportunity to identify other disabilities which might affect speech development.

Gross disorders such as cleft palate, blindness, and cerebral palsy are obvious. Neuromuscular incoordination, visual defects, and mental retardation may be revealed through testing or observation. Instructional experience is probably the only way to ascertain clues to milder but significant disabilities and to pervasive problems in language learning. The latter are often difficult to pinpoint and their precise definition is frequently elusive. A good illustration of this issue is the history of controversy surrounding the early identification of "congenital aphasia." Table 7 shows additional handicapping conditions encountered in schools and classes for the deaf as reported to the Office of Demographic Studies at Gallaudet College (124).

Of course, when combined with hearing loss, disabilities may retard or in extreme cases prevent the acquisition of speech—this despite excellence of teaching in the context of an environment that promotes its use. Nevertheless, it is irresponsible to assume *at the outset* that certain disabilities, of whatever degree or kind, will preclude learning to speak. Confident prediction of their precise effect is indeed precarious and difficult. The child should have the benefit of appropriate and sufficient empirical tests of assumptions about his ability to learn to talk. To do otherwise is to arrive at an all too common self-fulfilling prophecy. If a child is treated as though he will not learn, he will not learn.

4. The method should provide sufficient experience for assessing progress in speech development.

Knowledge of a child's previous experience with intervention for speech development can influence not only initial steps but also the efficacy of continuing with the previous approach or of changing to an alternate one. Specifically we should know the nature and duration of the experience and the progress in speech or speech-like behavior resulting from it. Two 30-month-old children with similar hearing levels cannot be compared for speech development when one has worn a hearing aid for 12 months and the other not at all, or when one has had guidance in his home environment through an early education program and the other has only been fitted with a hearing aid and given no treatment. Chapter II addresses itself to ways to describe the nature of the child's experience.

In addition to the total time elapsed from beginning to end of the experience, the amount of time during which the child has been directly involved warrants attention. The duration of an experience that will influence the decision about change in approach is likely to vary with chronological age. The older the child the less time there is available for observing the progress resulting from initial procedures. Nevertheless, sufficient time should be allowed to make a reasonably confident judgment.

We are usually inclined to compare the young child's speech output with that of normal children of the same chronological age or with that of other deaf children of a similar age and hearing level. We may compare the rate of speech development and the amount, spontaneity, and intelligibility of speech. But when the child has had previous intervention, we should assess his speech production before and after that experience, comparing his progress with that of similar children who have undergone the same experience.

It is our considered judgment that the above requirements are best met by the Auditory Global method and we recommend it as the initial method of choice. Realistically we need to anticipate that the Auditory Global method will not be satisfactory for all children. Careful regular assessment of the child's progress in learning to talk is essential as suggested by this simple flow chart.

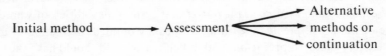

ASSESSMENT

Time for Assessment

With the initial approach, no hard and fast rules can be laid down for the best length of experience or for the age of the child before formal speech assessment, but Table 12 provides some general guidelines. A two- to three-year

Age at Beginning of Initial Approach	Age at Assessment
6 months	2 to 3 years
1 to 2 years	3 to 4 years
3 to 4 years	4 to 5 years
5 years	5.5 to 6 years
6 years	6.5 years

Table 12.   Guide to term of initial approach and age at assessment.

period of experience with the initial approach gives a reasonably good opportunity to judge a very young child's progress. On the other hand, by the time he is of kindergarten age it is important to have him placed in the kind of program he will find to best advantage. Regardless of age, though, the initial approach experience should probably not be less than six months. Even before the formal assessment takes place, the teacher and parents should have been making continuous observations during the experience which will be helpful to gauge the child's progress.

Questions for Assessment

After a reasonable experience with the Auditory Global method, assessment should address three basic questions:
1. What progress has the child made in speech development?
2. What special problems does the child have in learning speech?
3. Can an environment conducive to speech development be maintained?

1. What Progress Has the Child Made in Speech Development?

Progress in speech development should consider the aspects of speech discussed in previous chapters, **voice, rhythm,** and **articulation.** Now ready for assessment is speech **usage,** an additional important dimension. If the child is making good progress with the Auditory Global method, the volume of his voice should be adequate to carry speech to the average listener and his voice quality should approximate that of a child of his age with normal hearing. The normal temporal features and intonation of connected speech, fundamental outcomes of the Auditory Global method, should be emerging. These include patterning of questions, declarative sentences, exclamations, and serial words. Arhythmic speech, as evidenced by single words serving as the total utterance, or words in the same phrase but separated by pauses and having undifferentiated syllabic value, suggests the need for change in method.

Articulation development should be well along. However, at an early age precise articulation is not critical. The Auditory Global method does not stress precision in the early years. The child should have many words recognizable at least to parents and teachers, rather than a few words accurately pronounced. Vowel/consonant differentiation should be made easily. Manner and/or place of articulation along with coarticulation should be approximated or achieved. A pertinent question here is whether the child has formed an abstract phonological system similar to that of a normal talker. For example, in addition to emerging manner and place features, does the child produce normal durational differences resulting from phonetic context? Consider the duration of the vowels **ee** and **-i-** in the words *eat* and *ease,* and in *it* and *is.* Note the difference in duration of the same vowels determined by the consonant following. To assess articulation at this time, a picture description test which demands **connected speech** may be more useful than a single-word picture-naming test, but a combination of the two should not be ruled out.

In most situations, the child should be using speech to make his wants known, to respond to others, and to initiate communication. The utterances are likely to be accompanied by gestures just as with a normal child. Of course, semantic and syntactic development of spoken language should be noted. A promising guide for judging them is the Scales of Early Communication Skills for Hearing Impaired Children developed by Moog and Geers at Central Institute for the Deaf. These Scales appear in the Appendix.

2. What Special Problems Does the Child Have in Learning Speech?

A reasonable amount of experience should reveal to the alert teacher any special problems in learning speech. The handicapping effects of obvious disabilities, such as vision or motor control and others listed in Table 7, can be assessed. If a special problem in learning speech exists, change to another method may be indicated to accommodate that problem. Of course the child's progress, despite the disability, must be considered.

3. Can an Environment Conducive to Speech Development Be Maintained?

In Chapter II we outlined the requirements for an "oral environment," and earlier in this chapter we have stressed the need for comprehensive support for communication in the child's home and community. The parents' attitudes and interest in working with their child and in cooperating with the professionally directed program may influence the decision to discontinue the Auditory Global method, even though the child has the potential for benefiting from it. For example, the professional staff may note that, despite counseling and reminders, the parents have not kept the child's hearing aid constantly operative, have not made and kept appointments for hearing examinations as advised, or have not provided speech stimulation. An impoverished auditory-oral environment, whatever its cause, will render ineffective the Auditory Global method.

If assessment of experience with the Auditory Global method is judged to be satisfactory we recommend its continuance beyond the preschool, keeping in mind the previously mentioned pragmatic points that need to be considered. Among the conventional options to accomplish this are:

a. No special assistance: One alternative is to place the hearing impaired child in a regular class with no provision for special assistance. This assumes that auditory stimulation in the natural course of events will be sufficient to maintain continuing speech development; it is indicated generally for those children with moderate degrees of hearing loss who use hearing aids very effectively. Guidance for the parents and classroom teacher may be necessary to ensure a facilitating acoustic environment. Periodic reassessment should include an analysis of hearing, electroacoustic measurements of the characteristics of the hearing aid, and, of course, evaluation of speech and language development. Lagging speech development may call for more intensive procedures.

b. Special tutorial assistance: Some children will require the support of tutorial assistance that supplements their placement in a regular full-time classroom. Such assistance may be obtained through the school speech and hearing program, from a community agency, or through a private tutor. The speech tutor should have the dual responsibility to foster speech development and to maintain maximal auditory stimulation through auditory training. For such a child speech deviations are likely to be articulatory, although voice and rhythm may require some attention. Here and there some special language instruction may be included in the supportive regimen.

c. Part- or full-time special class: A third alternative is to enroll the child in a special class part of his school day, providing regular classes the rest of the day. This situation should include a program of parental guidance, guidance for teachers of those regular classes in which the child is enrolled, and annual reassessment of hearing, of hearing aids, and of speech and language development. The special class should provide intensive communication instruction and assistance with other academic instruction. It may range from a resource room which the child attends for only one hour a day to a special class for most or all of the day.

The program should be flexible enough to enable a child to move from one to the other of these situations. Children commonly termed "mildly hard of hearing," "moderately hard of hearing," "moderately deaf," or "deaf" may be included. Such terms are irrelevant. The child's academic achievement, his social development, and his progress in language and speech—rather than his hearing level—should be the deciding factors.

If progress by the Auditory Global method is judged to be unsatisfactory, then we recommend either the Multisensory Syllable Unit method or the Association Phoneme Unit method. Our choice between these two methods depends upon assessment of experience that addresses itself to the same questions posed for the Auditory Global method. Obviously the answers to these questions need to take into account the child's age and the reasonableness of the length of experience.

What progress has the child made in speech development? In general this child requires multisensory stimulation to develop speech. Assessment, therefore, should focus on how the child responds to such stimulation. He should be able to respond by imitation to vibro-tactile and visual cues that may convey speech information about place, manner, voicing, duration, pitch, loudness, and patterning. Of course, auditory stimulation should always be available. Retention and retrieval of stored phonologic information should be demonstrated. Depending on the child's stage of development, this may be elicited by pointing to an orthographic symbol, a picture, or a written word or phrase. There should be evidence of the ability to produce increasingly longer combinations of segments of speech without abnormal motor effort. As the child learns orthographic symbols, he should be strengthening his power to attack the production of new vocabulary graphically presented—for example, oral reading of chart language. Fundamentally, as with the Auditory Global method, speech should be developing as a vehicle for everyday communication, initiated by the child and not perceived by him merely as a classroom gymnastic.

By this time the retarding effects of the kinds of special problems cited during the early Auditory Global method period will have been noted. It is important, too, that a continuing reinforcing oral environment be maintained and that the child's teachers be skilled in multisensory methods. If the assessment leads to a reasonably positive judgment, the Multisensory Syllable Unit method should be used. If not, the Association Phoneme Unit method should be tried with the expectancy that the child can "graduate" to one or the other of the methods, or a combination of them.

From what we have said about choosing among methods, it is evident that although exclusive, incontrovertibly valid techniques for making decisions are not immediately at hand, there are sufficient bases for making rational judgments. Furthermore, we repeat that sensible management requires periodic evaluation and that one should avoid an attitude of irrevocable commitment to a particular method. The possibility of shift in method or of employing effective combinations of methods should always be kept in mind.

CHAPTER VI

Beyond Development of Speech

In this chapter we shall assume that the foundation for speech development, as treated in Chapter V, has been laid. We now turn our attention to the instructional activities that build upon it and lead to improvement. As we have said in the Introduction, speech must not only be developed; it must be improved, corrected, and maintained. It is difficult, and perhaps not too helpful, to attempt a fine delineation among the goals of improvement, correction, and maintenance. Here and there in this chapter we shall emphasize implicitly one or the other, but—realistically—instructional procedures are likely to be a blend of all three and even include development. It is probable that the speech of deaf children may improve with usage and in response to social demands made upon them to communicate, but this is not likely to happen—particularly during school age—without planned intervention that derives from a child's individual speech program that is carefully thought-out. De-emphasis of speech instruction as a child advances through the grades not only risks the detrimental effect on acquired competence but also devalues its importance for him.

In general, improvement centers not only on specifically targeted aspects of articulation, voice, and rhythm, but also on closing the gap between performance in the disciplined context of speech instruction and in the everyday situation of oral exchange, frequently referred to as the "carry-over." For example, in the disciplined context the child typically produces units or

173

segments clearly superior to his production in less organized situations. This stresses the need for alertness of the teacher in recognizing and responding to a child's capabilities. Furthermore, the quality of speech production when induced by the teacher is likely to be better than when the child uses spontaneously initiated speech. We must keep in mind that in communicating orally the child must not only attend to the phonology of his message, he must also give thought to its semantic and syntactic requirements. This complex task may reduce the care with which his demonstrated ability in the production of single or small units is incorporated in flowing utterances.

Sensitivity and responsiveness of the teacher—and for that matter of all who are responsible for a child's development—to the need for carry-over should strengthen the child's confidence in his speech as a socially significant skill. This is necessary to foster, if not actually to determine, its social usefulness. We are less likely to avoid a task if we have confidence in our ability to perform it. Of course, in our efforts to expand the opportunities for speech usage, we must caution against shattering a child's confidence by placing him in situations where his failure to be understood may demoralize him. He benefits from practice in social situations with sympathetic listeners who may inform him tactfully that they do not understand but who give him an opportunity to "reach back" for the best performance of which he is capable.

Essential to the improvement of speech is the correction of deviations. Correction may require teacher-initiated measures or self-correction by the talker, but usually a combination of both. We shall deal first with the teacher's part.

The teacher needs to maintain a continuing, but not overly intrusive, attitude of awareness of the **deviation from acceptable speech**. Acceptability will vary with the state of speech competence of the talker. Here the teacher will need to take into account the expectancies for each individual child. The teacher's observation of deviations in a child's speech should guide the development of his individual program. She should not depend solely on her "daily running assessment" but should make a periodic organized assessment which will lead to planned measures for correction.

Improvement and correction of speech, whether in response to its production in the variety of situations that occur in daily activities or in purposeful structured drills, can be conceptualized around an ordered sequence of the kind described in Chapter II in our discussion of methodology. The first steps in the sequence are likely to be more applicable in unstructured situations, the later steps more pertinent for work in "speech periods."

Signaling

The teacher conventionally signals an error, abnormality, or irregularity by some expression such as, "What did you say?" or, "I did not understand you." Facial expressions, even raising the eyebrows, frequently constitute signaling.

Specifying

Specification is achieved on a gradient ranging from the initial signal which may be ineffective to accomplish correction to a clearly specified particular deviation. The aim throughout is to avoid a uniform "style" of specification of deviation and to achieve talker self-correction, by his recall, whenever possible. Specification may be oral, written, or both. The progression along the gradient, with illustrative teacher responses, could go something like this:

1. *Communicate the locus of the deviation.* "I didn't understand the first part of your sentence."
2. *Indicate the type of deviation.*
   a. *Indicate* that a combination of phonemes or a single one is in error without identification. "You left out a sound."
   b. *Indicate* a voice abnormality. "Watch your voice."
   c. *Indicate* a rhythmic irregularity. "You forgot the accents."
3. *Identify the point of deviation.*
   a. *Identify* the phoneme or combination. "You can say **ch** better in ____."
   b. *Identify* voice abnormality. "I could not hear you."
   c. *Identify* rhythmic irregularity. "The accent in ____ should be on the first, not the second syllable."
4. *Describe the nature of the error* (this applies to articulation). "You said **b** through your nose."

The remaining items in the sequence require more active participation by the teacher.

Correcting

1. *Model the desired speech orally for the child to imitate.* The model should avoid exaggerated articulation or tension, either deliberate or unconscious.
2. *Demonstrate over whatever sensory channels and mode best accomplish the communication of the abnormality and its correction.*

   a. A useful paradigm is to communicate the child's deviation by exaggerating it and then to exaggerate in the desired direction of correction. For example, if the child seems to insert a superfluous neutral vowel between **ee** and **l** in *meal*, then the teacher may give a full-length vowel between the two

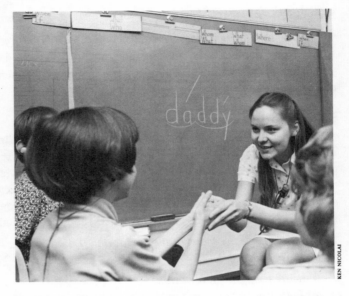

Clapping the hands to develop appreciation for accent.

sounds as illustration of what not to do and, for correction, give a voiceless **l** even though some voicing is required.

b. Use easily perceived analogies. For example, excessive or inadequate pressure for plosives may be indicated by pressing the thumb in the palm of the hand or blowing a strip of paper. Rhythm may be shown by tapping on the shoulder or clapping the hands.

c. In cases of poor visibility or audibility it may be necessary to depart from natural production to communicate, for example, place of articulation. The demonstration of a lingua-velar **k** in the combination **koo** would require opening the mouth wider than necessary in order to make the articulation visible. Care should be taken to avoid this as a recurring model which is likely to produce speech with inordinate pervasive jaw movement. If in a two-syllable word like *mother* equal stress is given to both syllables, a very loud first syllable and an almost voiceless second syllable may be helpful.

d. Discriminate among abnormalities that are class-like—whether of manner, place, etc.—and those that are specific to a particular sound. Excessive pressure may be characteristic of all plosives, or lingua-dental positions may reveal inadequate control of the tip of the tongue. Demonstrations should, therefore, include all members of a class and lead to generalization.

e. Reduce phonetic complexity by demonstrating a sound out of context to focus attention on it. Affricates like **ch** frequently need concentrated demonstration of the relation between the stop and fricative components. Of course, the sound then needs to be demonstrated in a variety of phonetic contexts.

f. Demonstrate by whatever sensory aids are available and applicable (see Chapter II).

3. *Manipulate the speech mechanism.* This involves shaping accessible parts of the speech mechanism—rounding the lips, pressing the tongue down or forcing it up—all to achieve motor action or accurate placement. It should be a last resort in correcting.

DEVIATIONS OF SPEECH

Experience has demonstrated, at least by instructional methods employed up to the present, that certain deviations are likely to occur frequently enough to warrant checking for them in any formal assessment. The conventional way of assessing for deviations is to attend to spontaneous speech and to elicit devised samples from written items, picture descriptions, or combinations of these. In the sense that a physician looks for common symptoms, diseases, and causes, the teacher bases her assessment on the possible errors of articulation, abnormalities of voice, and irregularities of rhythm described in this chapter as well as on the review of individual phonemes in Chapter IV. These judgments will depend on the child's stage of speech and language development. In planning remedial measures the teacher needs to distinguish whether a deviation is a failure to carry over a skill that a child already possesses or whether the skill needs to be acquired or possibly improved. Failure to carry over—generally observed in connected speech—whether spontaneous or elicited, suggests that the teacher simply remind the child about the deviation according to the sequence presented earlier in this chapter. Acquisition and improvement require planned intervention. The reader is referred to Chapter IV for suggestions for remediation of specific articulatory errors of omission, substitution, distortion, and addition.

The following catalogue of possible deviations is definitely not all-inclusive. The teacher's *power of analysis* should be brought to bear on any deviation.

Errors of Articulation

In Chapter IV we described errors in the production of individual phonemes and their correction. In table 13 we have rank ordered groups of phonemes on a scale of frequency of need for correction as judged by teachers at Central Institute for the Deaf. It is interesting to note the substantial agreement with the study by Hudgins and Numbers at the Clarke and Pennsylvania Schools for the Deaf. It is probable that the children in these studies were taught by what we have called the Multisensory Syllable Unit method.

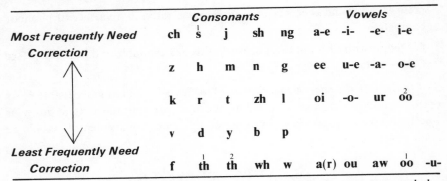

	Consonants					Vowels				
Most Frequently Need Correction	ch	$\overset{1}{s}$	j	sh	ng	a-e	-i-	-e-	i-e	
	z	h	m	n	g	ee	u-e	-a-	o-e	
	k	r	t	zh	l	oi	-o-	ur	$\overset{2}{oo}$	
	v	d	y	b	p					
Least Frequently Need Correction	f	$\overset{1}{th}$	$\overset{2}{th}$	wh	w	a(r)	ou	aw	$\overset{1}{oo}$	-u-

Table 13. Rank ordering of phonemes by frequency of correction needed.

Errors of articulation are not confined to production of individual phonemes. They can and do occur because of the phonetic context in which the phonemes are imbedded. A child may be able to produce a perfect $\overset{1}{s}$ in isolation but may omit or distort it in flowing speech. Furthermore, errors may be of a large-class or subclass variety. A large-class error may be voice-voiceless confusion that may reveal itself in a number of phonemes. Production of affricates may be a subclass error, as in the release of the **k** in the word *six* resulting in the intrusion of a neutral vowel between the **k** and $\overset{1}{s}$ and producing a listener set for a two-syllable word. Furthermore, multiple causes may lead to single effects and single causes may lead to multiple effects, as we shall see in what follows.

1. Errors of Omission

a. Omission of $\overset{1}{s}$ in all contexts: Because it is both a frequently occurring phoneme and one that is often omitted, we have singled out $\overset{1}{s}$ for emphasis. As we have seen in Table 4, $\overset{1}{s}$ ranks low in internal feedback, and its poor visibility limits the child's exposure to it. It has been noted that omission of $\overset{1}{s}$ is a prominent deviation in the speech of the adult whose hearing is failing.

b. Omission of the final consonant: Omission of final consonants by young deaf children is sometimes caused by forgetting to articulate the consonant, but in older speakers, the apparent omission of final consonants is more likely to be caused by one or more of three conditions of articulation distortion. These are:

(1) Reduced force on arresting consonants,

(2) Lack of coarticulation effect on preceding vowels, and

(3) Abnormal duration of the preceding vowels in relation to the final consonants.

In the syllable with an arresting consonant, important acoustic information about the consonant is conveyed by the duration of the vowel and its formant transitions (spectral changes as the vowel moves toward the consonant). When the vowel is longer than it should be and "trails off" in expended energy, the listener is misled by the wrong cue. If in the word *beet* the **ee** is prolonged and the effects of coarticulation are lost as it trails off, the listener does not anticipate the final stop and judges that it is absent. When these effects are combined with reduced force on the final consonant, particularly on stops but not confined to them, it appears that the consonant has been omitted.

An instance of consonant omission worthy of mention is **ng** as in the word *sing*. This apparent omission is frequently caused by the production of **ng** with insufficient opening of the nasopharyngeal port. The **ng** sounds like a continuation of the preceding vowel.

c. Omission of initial consonants: A consonant initiating a syllable may be perceived to have been omitted when it is distorted by reduced force. Plosive consonants are often released with insufficient force for the listener either to perceive its presence or to use the cue of the coarticulation effect on the formant transitions of the following vowel. Reduced force on the stop breath consonants **p, t,** and **k** also reduces their duration, and the listener may confuse them with their voiced cognates **b, d,** and **g,** or may even fail to perceive that they have been said at all.

2. Errors of Substitution

When the deaf child is developing speech, he is likely to have several consonant substitutions, much like the child with normal hearing who has not yet mastered the phonologic rules underlying spoken language. As he grows older these substitutions tend to diminish. Those remaining substitutions, some apparent, some real, are likely to be distorted productions of the intended consonants by the speaker, heard as different consonants by the listener.

a. Voice-breath consonant substitutions: An error considered uniquely typical of deaf speakers is the "surd-sonant," or the substitution of one sound for another when the sounds have the same place of articulation but differ in the voice-voiceless feature. Thus the breath (surd) stop consonant **p** may be heard as its voiced (sonant) stop consonant cognate **b,** or the reverse. Other cognates which are frequently confused are **t** and **d, k** and **g, f** and **v,** and **th** and **th**.

As with the apparent omission of consonants, the substitution of these cognates for each other may be caused by articulation distortion. When a vowel precedes a breath consonant, for example, some deaf speakers continue the voice into the consonant. The resulting acoustic information suggests substitution of the voiced cognate of the intended breath consonant. Similarly, voicing for the following vowel may begin before the breath consonant has been completed, giving the listener voiced consonant information. Initiating and terminating voicing requires exquisite timing. In addition, as we pointed out previously, the surd-sonant error may have its roots in the inappropriate force of consonant articulation or in the abnormal duration of associated vowels (**eet-eed**).

Our observations indicate that the surd-sonant error is not the simple substitution of one sound for another. It is an error of distortion by the deaf talker which influences the perception for the listener. In summary the causes of the distortion appear to be:

(1) Inadequate coordination of voicing and articulation. This point is supported by the ease with which deaf talkers can produce cognates accurately in isolation;

(2) Inappropriate force of articulation causing duration distortion of the consonant; and

(3) Distortion of the duration of vowels preceding consonants.

b. Nasal-oral consonant substitution: A nasal consonant may be substituted for its oral cognate (**m** for **b**, **n** for **d**, and **ng** for **g**). Deaf speakers, unlike hearing persons with palatal insufficiency, also reverse the substitution, so we have **b** for **m**, **d** for **n**, **g** for **ng**. Here again the nasal-oral consonant substitution rests primarily on improper coordination, in this case of the nasopharyngeal closure. Compounding of surd-sonant and oral-nasal errors may result in **m** substituted for the breath **p**, **n** for **t**, and **ng** for **k**.

c. Low feedback substitutions: Production of some sounds is likely to provide little sensory feedback, while the substituted sound provides more perceivable feedback, especially tactile. For example, **w** or **l** may be substituted for **r**. The vocalized continuing nature of the consonant is appropriate, but the speaker seeks better feedback than a typical **r** provides. With the substituted **w** the speaker monitors the production from the kinesthetic impression of lip rounding. With the substituted **l** the tactile impression is strong for the tip of the tongue touching the palate.

Similarly **t** or **th** may be substituted for the low feedback **s**. The speaker seeks tactile feedback by touching the tongue and alveolar ridge for **t**, or seeks increased perception of friction by producing a **th**.

d. Vowel substitutions: The apparent substitution of vowels is caused largely by imprecision. As we have seen in Chapter I, exceedingly fine differences of mouth opening, rounding of lips, and place and height of tongue arching are required for accurate vowel formation. The differences among vowels give very little tactile or kinesthetic feedback. The vowel perceived is most likely to be one which adjoins the vowel intended, as represented on the vowel diagram (Figure 7). A common vowel substitution, for example, would be -e- for -a- with the listener hearing *met* for the intended *mat*. The speaker is not likely to substitute a vowel with lip rounding (oͪo) for one without rounding (ee).

3. Errors of Distortion

a. Degree of force: Stop and fricative consonants are frequently made with either too much or too little force. Too little force gives the listener acoustic information of abnormally shortened duration and reduced intensity. He may hear the sound as a distortion of the intended consonant or as another consonant, or may sense the absence of an expected sound. Too much force gives the listener acoustic information of abnormally long duration and increased intensity. He may hear a distorted or a substituted consonant.

A frequent source of distortion is excessive force in producing stops **p, t, k, b, d,** and **g**. For example, **p** and **t** are often distorted by too much bilabial or lingua-alveolar pressure combined with excessive jaw movement. This may lead to breathiness of a following vowel as the residual air at the glottal sound source is insufficient to produce the vowel, or to diphthongization of the vowel as the jaw is returned to the required mouth opening.

b. Hypernasality: Deaf speakers, who experience difficulty with the fine coordination of rapid oral/nasal resonance changes in connected speech, produce hypernasal sounds. Consonants **b, d,** and **g** may be heard as substituted sounds **m, n,** and **ng**. Consonants **l, r, w, v, th,** and **z**, too, may be mistaken for one of the nasal consonants **m, n,** or **ng**, or may give the impression of a distorted and often non-targeted, indistinguishable sound. Nasal consonants may cause nasalization of the preceding or following vowel. In the syllable **ṃa(r)**, the **a(r)** may be nasalized if the speaker fails to return the velum to its required position for vowel production. Vowels associated with a nasal consonant are vulnerable to nasalization particularly when the air flow to the oral cavity is restricted by the closeness of the velum and back of the tongue. High vowels oͪo and **ee** are examples of this.

The nasalization of certain vowels and consonants and their combinations should not be confused with pervasive abnormality of voice in which all voiced speech sounds are nasalized. As we shall see later, such nasalization is a general difficulty of voice production.

c. Imprecision and indefiniteness: We recall from Chapters I and IV, and from our comments on substitutions, that vowels are produced by exquisitely slight variations in mouth opening, place and height of arching the tongue, and rounding of the lips. These variations in the vocal tract give rise to formant differences that constitute important, if not exclusive, listening cues. Deaf speakers may be slightly off target with respect to one or more of these required variations in the production of certain vowels, particularly those with low kinesthetic feedback. This applies especially to the front vowels **ee, -i-, -e-,** and **-a-** where lip rounding is not available as a monitoring production cue. On the other hand, some vowels are produced indefinitely and the listener has no class category cue at all. In the case of imprecision, **-i-** may be confused with **-e-,** and **-e-** with **-a-.** But the indefinite vowel is ambiguous for the listener. These observations apply also to vowel-like consonants **l, r, y,** and **w.**

d. *Duration of vowels:* The duration of vowels in connected speech should vary according to context. These systematic variations give the listener important acoustic cues to adjoining sounds. For example, vowels preceding voiceless consonants are typically shorter than the same vowels before voiced consonants (*beat-bead, leaf-leave*). The listener gets cues about the voicing and even identification of the consonant. Deaf speakers tend to produce vowels with undifferentiated duration. The tendency is likely to be in the direction of excessive duration (103).

e. *Temporal values in diphthongs:* Diphthongs combine two continuously phonated vowels, with the first portion (the nucleus) longer than the second (the glide), except for **u-e** where the relations are reversed. Deaf speakers may make the second portion longer than it needs to be. The effort to produce both elements accurately splits the diphthong, making two discrete vowels. *Buy* becomes **ba(r)-ee,** *tape* becomes **te-eep** and *house* becomes **ha(r)-us,** giving the listener a message set for a two-syllable word. The error in the other direction either reduces the length of the glide or eliminates it entirely—*bait* becomes **bet,** *night* becomes **na(r)t,** and *cloud* becomes **kla(r)d.** Drills on vowels need to develop awareness of variations in their durational features and time relations. "Sing-song" drills that produce vowels of uniform duration should be avoided. Unless otherwise indicated, as in the case of a small increment approach, syllable drills should be of the consonant-vowel-consonant (CVC) type.

4. *Errors of Addition*

a. *Insertion of a superfluous vowel between consonants:* Adjoining consonants occur in various relations to each other. Among the important combinations of interest to us are ***blends,*** where **l** and **r** are preceded by consonants and the position for **l** and **r** is taken before the first consonant is produced (*blue, try*); ***clusters*** (*snow*), particularly affricates (*looks*); and ***abutting consonants*** (*football*), where they occur adjacent to each other but in separate syllables.

In these combinations the deaf talker may insert a superfluous neutral vowel that sounds almost like a brief **-u-** and the listener gets a misleading syllabic cue. In the case of blends this may be caused either by failure to take the position of **l** or **r** before articulating the preceding consonant (*blue*-**bulóo**) or by voicing the **l** and **r** when preceded by a voiceless consonant (*try*-**turi-e**). In clusters the breath-voice sequence may be improperly coordinated and the voicing commenced in the transition from the breathed to the voiced consonant (*snow*-**suno-e**). In affricates the stop may be completely released with voicing before the fricative is given (*looks*-**lóokus**), and in the abutting consonants, too, the first consonant is released before the second consonant is given (*football*-**fóotubawl**, *good night*-**goodunite**).

b. Unnecessary release of final stop consonants: A distracting and frequently misleading insertion may be the forceful release of a final stop consonant as in "It's time to stop____," or "Go to bed____." The talker appears to have a static conception of the consonant produced in isolation and requires explosion at all times. Unfortunately, he may have been *taught* that this is the case.

c. Diphthongization of vowels: Certain vowel-consonant combinations require faster and smoother transitions than deaf talkers are likely to produce. Errors such as these result: *meat*-**meeut,** *feel*-**feeul,** *bed*-**beud,** *moon*-**móoun.** In **meeut,** for example, the transition of the movement of the tongue from the vowel to the lingua-alveolar position—from **ee** to **t**—is too slow, and voicing—again the brief **-u-** like sound—intrudes, giving rise to what appears to be a bisyllabic utterance.

d. Superfluous breath before a vowel: Vowels, of course, are all voiced. Deaf talkers, however, may precede a vowel by unnecessary aspiration, particularly a vowel that initiates an utterance. Apparently air is forcefully aspirated before the vocal folds approximate to produce phonation. The listener perceives the aspiration as an **h.** Incidentally, in combinations that require **h,** which always is produced in the position of the vowel that follows, the deaf talker may over-aspirate in a discrete position or he may omit the **h** as in cockney speech.

Abnormalities of Voice

It has been our observation that deviations in voice and irregularities of rhythm are posing less of a problem than heretofore, due perhaps to early application of the Auditory Global method. As we have seen, "errors" of articulation are reasonably specifiable, whereas abnormalities of voice require judgments that are generally expressed by adjectives that do not always mean the same to those who use them. This supports the generalization that the less a science has advanced, the more its terminology tends to rest upon the uncritical assumption of mutual understanding. Our experience suggests that even teachers tend to use a variety of terms about "deaf voices," generally negative in their connotation. It has been found that frequently used terms included *dull, hollow, raspy, piercing, tense, flat, breathy, harsh, throaty,* and *shrieking* (104). Never mentioned were terms such as *mellow, warm, smooth, full, vibrant, pear shaped,* or *clear.* For a penetrating review of parameters of voice quality, correlates of voice production, and a behavioral analysis of vocal function, the reader is referred to Chapters 17, 18, and 19 of the *Handbook of Speech Pathology and Audiology* (200).

Perhaps as useful a way as any to organize our presentation of abnormalities in voice is to discuss them in terms that are rather more descriptive of the observed vocal output than are some of the ambiguous adjectives mentioned above. These are *nasality, breathiness, stridency, inadequate loudness, fundamental pitch,* and *uncontrolled pitch.*

1. Nasality: We recall that English phonology includes only three nasal sounds, **m, n,** and **ng,** in which the nasopharyngeal port is open. Hypernasality, the opening of the port when not necessary for the utterance, is unfortunately a frequent condition of deaf talkers. It is interesting that in a cinefluorographic study comparing five typical deaf speakers producing oral syllables (not necessarily judged to be hypernasal) it was found that the experimental deaf group all exhibited velopharyngeal opening, which was not true of the normally-speaking control group (155). McClumpha found the deaf speakers to have shorter and thinner velums, which may result from lack of muscle activity involved in velopharyngeal closure and oral voice production. Of course, not to be overlooked as a cause of hypernasality may be an observable cleft or velar insufficiency.

When indicated, the improvement of voice—whether of nasality, breathiness, stridency, loudness, or pitch—should recognize the importance of conveying to the child what he is doing and what needs to be done. Sensory aids that display voice and rhythm parameters may be helpful and should be employed, but the alert ear of the teacher is still the major "error detector." The teacher must be able to imitate the child's deviation and to communicate it, frequently exaggerated, in order to give the child an unambiguous cue to the deviation. All principles of discriminating use of sensory channels, previously discussed, apply here. Trial and error invariably operate in the process of improving voice. The teacher needs to reinforce aggressively every satisfactory production. For hypernasality the child can feel the teacher's nose and the reduction of oral pressure. Exercises should concentrate on directing the breath stream through the oral cavity and giving the child the feel" of velopharyn-geal action. Just inhaling and exhaling through a wide open mouth and hold-ing the position can communicate a feel of the velar movement. Then com-bining a nasal consonant—such as **ng**—with a vowel, both given with force, can accomplish this. These should form the basis for more elaborate nasal/non-nasal combinations.

2. Breathiness: The vowels of English require alternating closure of the glottis by contact of the vocal folds without unnecessary leakage of air. The inefficient control of this process leads again to a distracting voice quality and may actually degrade intelligibility. The closure of the folds may be either in-complete or too brief, or both. The condition may be reflected prominently in abnormally short phrased speech separated by unnecessarily frequent in-halations, sometimes referred to as "pumping." Recall, too, the excessive force on plosives preceding a vowel that may give it a breathy quality.

Breathiness can be communicated by having the child feel excessive air at the mouth during the phonation of a vowel and, of course, in connected speech, followed by the teacher's model of proper phonation. A strip of paper in front of the mouth can be observed to yield to the air stream, too. Some-times a circle of moisture from the breath is visible on a chalk board or mir-ror. The child should try to produce vowels without bending the strip of pa-per, and he should also be required to count without taking a breath and continue to extend the number he attains by economizing on the use of air. For fluency, it should go "one-and-two-and-three-and-," etc. Holding a weight such as a stack of books, or pushing against a table while phonating, attains proper glottal action.

3. Stridency: The normal talker uses the muscles for articulation and voic-ing synergistically. The muscles "work together" without undue tension. Per-haps because he gropes for feedback or because he has been taught with over-emphasis on the tactile impression gained from feeling a teacher's larynx, the deaf talker may speak with a great deal of generalized constriction and ten-sion in both the glottal and supraglottal areas. The result is commonly termed stridency or, by some, harshness. Of course the teacher in her determination to develop good speech must be mindful to avoid tension in the model she presents to children.

The teacher can demonstrate stridency by letting the child feel her exagger-ated muscle tension just above the larynx in saying a vowel and then feel the change that comes with return to normal muscle action. The child should not be expected to imitate the teacher's voice. He should be imitating her muscle action in those muscles that are accessible for demonstration. At times the bunching of the tongue in the back of the mouth needs to be explored and the child should be directed and shown to keep his tongue forward. When satisfactory production for a vowel has been achieved, additional vowels should be tried and then combined with sequences of familiar expressions.

4. *Loudness:* Normal talkers regulate loudness to accommodate to distance from a listener, to requirements of social situations, and to varying levels of ambient noise. Deaf talkers may be unaware of these conditions or may simply not be able to speak loud enough in any situation. Inefficient use of the air stream at the glottis may be responsible for the inability to speak loud enough. The suggestions for remediation of breathiness apply here.

5. *Fundamental pitch:* Both young male and young female deaf talkers tend to speak with a higher fundamental pitch than hearing persons with whom they have been matched in controlled investigations (128). In another acoustic analysis, Calvert (103) not only confirmed the higher fundamental frequency but also observed that deaf talkers exhibited a smaller separation of the fundamental frequency (higher than normal) and the first formant of the vowel -a- (lower than normal). While this higher fundamental pitch for deaf speakers may not interfere with intelligibility, it may intrude a characteristic that adds to listener effort. The higher fundamental pitch may be particularly noticeable for young adult deaf speakers when it should be getting lower as they grow older.

6. *Pitch control:* Control of pitch relates to reasonable maintenance of range of the fundamental pitch of a particular talker, and of the deliberate variations in pitch that express speaker intent and satisfy the linguistic requirements of stress—whether of accent or intonation. The lack of control of fundamental pitch by deaf talkers results in distracting random and wide fluctuations. This condition is frequently associated with high arched vowels. The upward movement of the tongue raises the larynx and may over-tense the vocal folds, like stretching a rubber band.

As in the case of stridency, deviations in fundamental pitch generally grow out of improper muscle action not suited to the particular physiological mechanism of a talker. The manner of communication to the child and the remediation suggested for stridency apply here. The ability to control pitch and to apply it to linguistic requirements and talker intent are interrelated and will be treated under irregularities of rhythm.

Irregularities of Rhythm

In Chapter I we discussed the aspects of speech that contribute to its rhythm growing out of the syllabic patterning of accent, emphasis, intonation, phrasing, and rate. The rhythmic features are achieved by appropriate coarticulation and by controlled variations of loudness, pitch, and duration, especially of the vowel components of syllables. Irregularities of rhythm in the speech of deaf persons appear to have their origins in the difficulty of a talker to control the mechanics of varying loudness, pitch, and duration; and even if the skills have been fairly well achieved, the talker may not know when to apply them to communicate the intent of his message or to satisfy its linguistic requirements. The examples of irregularities, cited in Chapter I, are pertinent to the speech of deaf talkers. These views are underlined by Hood, who observed that deaf speakers used about two-thirds as much variation in fundamental frequency, one-half as much variation in intensity, extended syllable duration more than twice that of normal speakers, and syllabic values which seemed to be monotonously uniform (131). Irregular rhythm not only may be esthetically unappealing but also affects intelligibility significantly. Hudgins and Numbers (42) and Hood (131) found a high correlation for both normal and deaf speakers between intelligibility and judgments of rhythmic quality.

As we have seen in Chapter I, a symbol system to indicate rhythmic parameters is helpful. Many are used, but there should be consistency within a program. The symbols should indicate pitch, loudness, duration, and phrasing. An example of such a system, illustrated below, uses a horizontal line above syllables to suggest loudness (height) and duration (length), and a curving line to indicate pitch glides. A connecting line beneath a phrase could indicate its limits, and the number of slash marks would be a cue to length of pause.

$$\overline{} \quad \underline{}\,\overline{} \quad \underline{} \quad \underline{} \nearrow \quad \underline{}\,\overline{} \quad \overline{} \quad \underline{}\,\overline{} \nearrow \qquad \overline{}$$

Yesterday was a beautiful day / but today // it's terrible.

Although we have speculated that early intervention may reduce irregularities of rhythm, it is useful here to treat the process of its improvement. When satisfactory fundamental pitch has been achieved, pitch change to three or four levels on single vowels should be demonstrated, in ways previously discussed, and imitated by the child. Then, high and low vowels should be combined and given with controlled fundamental pitch and then with variations. Some suggested combinations are:

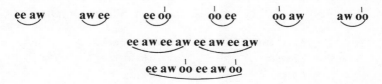

These should be followed by nonsense syllables and then by familiar expressions incorporating loudness and duration variations. Phrasing is aided by proper joining of words within phrases as well as by appropriate pauses. The following sentence, conventionally marked for phrasing, illustrates the point. "I don't think I can // but I want to try." The joining symbol ⌣ instructs the child to join the final sound of each word with the initial sound of the next word throughout the phrase. For example, the "I don't ---" is joined as though it were written "Idon't---"; the vowel **i-e** continues voicing as the position for **d** is taken. The sentence may also be marked for phrasing by using a continuous curved line under the entire phrase thus: "I don't think I can // but I want to try."

Consonants and vowels in adjoining words are joined in this example as follows:

"I don't think I can // but I want to try."

I don't — voicing on the vowel **i-e** continues as the position **d** is taken.
don't think — the stop consonant **t** is imploded and released into the position for **th,** as the tongue tip moves from the alveolar ridge to the edge of the upper teeth.
think I — **k i-e** blend is accomplished as though the **k** were the first sound of the syllable **ki-e.** To show this, the teacher may write the words in this fashion: "thing ki-e." Some teachers recommend that all syllables in a phrase be spoken with an initial consonant, even if the consonant is borrowed from the previous word.
I can — the vowel **i-e** is terminated by closure for the **k** stop consonant; the **n** is terminated by a pause.
but I — the **t i-e** blend is accomplished as though the final **t** of *but* were the first sound of the syllable **ti-e.**
I want — the **i-e** voicing continues as position is taken for the **w** and then the **aw,** almost like a triphthong.
want to — the abutting **t** sounds are blended into a single **t** sound which initiates the final syllable **too.**
to try — the vowel **oo** is terminated by closure for the **t** stop consonant in *try.*

On common short phrases, the teacher may demonstrate the joining of all phonemes, regardless of where words begin and end, by writing the phonemes of the phrase as though they were just one word. Some examples:

My name is	**mi-enameiz**
I live in	**i-elivin**
I am a	**i-eamu.**

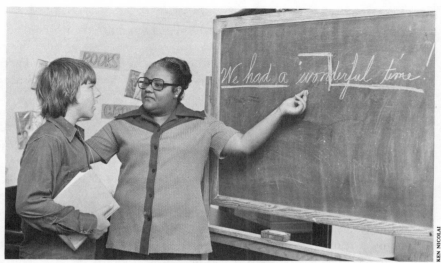

Coding patterns of speech.

Accent on appropriate syllables within words and emphasis on appropriate words within phrases and sentences are best achieved through increases in the force or stress with which the accented syllable or emphasized word is uttered. This may be shown to the child by writing the syllable or word to be stressed in bold, large capital letters, as in the following examples:

PUM pum	pum pum **PUM**
BAby	**CAN**dy
you **ARE** the one.	I want to go **NOW.**

Also useful are stress marks, such as the following:

púm pum	pum pum pum
báby	cándy
You are the one.	I want to go nów.

The teacher may also choose to underline words to be emphasized, as in the following examples:

You <u>are</u> the one.	I want to go <u>now</u>.

In all of the suggested exercises children should also be required to offer from their own repertoire matching linguistic patterns. For example, the teacher should ask the child to think of a pattern like "**CAN**dy." The patterns and uses of accents and emphasis were described in Chapter I.

In attempting increased force of articulation, the child is likely to make a change primarily in the loudness of his voice. Some increase in pitch will also result from increased force, but it may be best to emphasize only the increased loudness caused by the increased force in teaching stress production to the child.

Chapter I contains examples of linguistic requirements of English and patterns of speech that convey speaker intent. These form the basis for exercises in improvement of rhythm.

It is important to emphasize that although factors influencing the intelligibility of speech are treated differentially they are very much interrelated. Over-articulation can definitely contribute to abnormal voice quality and to irregular rhythm. An experiment by Calvert (104) relevant to this point is worthy of mention here. Experienced teachers of deaf children who were confident that they could identify a speaker as being deaf by just hearing his speech listened to samples from deaf speakers, normal speakers, speakers simulating deaf speech, and a person with a voice disorder. When the listeners heard only a steady voice cut from the center of a vowel sound, they could not tell accurately whether the speaker was deaf or hearing. As the articulatory complexity of the samples increased, the listeners became more accurate, reaching their highest accuracy on whole sentences. Table 14 shows the percentage of deaf and normal speech samples which met a 70% criterion of correct identification by a group of experienced teachers. It appears that as the deaf speaker moves through articulatory strings he gives the listener speech information that identifies him as a deaf speaker. It is likely that characteristics of articulation and rhythm, as well as voice quality, have led to identification of "deaf speech."

MAINTENANCE OF SPEECH

Throughout this book our emphasis has been properly and understandably on the speech of children. The general considerations, principles, methods, analyses, and activities all combine to maintain speech. It is important, however, to concern ourselves with post-school maintenance of speech where conventional organized programs are not available or feasible. We need to prepare children for this situation and advise adults no longer in school. We make the following suggestions to accomplish this:

1. Constant usage: There is no substitute for continual use of speech in all situations, not only to practice self-correction but also to reinforce confidence in its value.

2. Maximum use of amplification: As we have stressed for children, the adult should maintain and use the best possible acoustic amplification. Hear-

Speech Complexity Level	Accuracy Percentage
Cut vowels (center portion)	48%
Whole simple vowels	65%
Whole diphthongs	85%
CVC syllables	85%
CVCVC bisyllables	93%
Whole sentences	100%

Table 14. Percentage of deaf and normal speech samples meeting the criterion of 70% agreement at several levels of articulatory complexity.

ing and hearing aid evaluation should be carried out periodically by professionally qualified persons, and promising new hearing aids should be tried.

3. Awareness of speaking situations: A deaf person can help his naive listener in a number of ways. Among these are:

a. *Helping the listener to lipread.* In any stressful listening situation, whether because of ambient noise, competing messages, or deviant speech of a talker, the listener seeks supplementary visual cues. The deaf talker should place himself in a position so that his face is clearly visible.

b. *Helping the listener to hear.* Develop sensitivity to the requirements of the acoustic situation frequently, but not always, detectable by a hearing aid. The masking effects of noise, of whatever origin, and the influence of distance from the listener should be understood. If it is necessary and practical, a quiet place should be sought for conversation.

4. Preparing the listener: The listener can be helped and even put at ease if at the outset he is given a sample of "small talk" such as, "I'm glad to meet you," "How are you?" or "Good morning."

5. A second chance: When a listener does not understand speech, a deaf speaker should not assume that the listener understood *none* of what was said. He probably understood part but not enough to "put the pieces together" for complete understanding. The item should be repeated with *exactly* the words as first spoken. The listener will have a second chance to fill in what was first missed. Of course, if the listener does not understand the repeated sentence, the speaker must change the wording and resort to intentional redundancy. Here is a situation where economy of verbalization should not apply. Of course, as we have mentioned previously, the talker should make use of his internalized catalogue of "error probabilities."

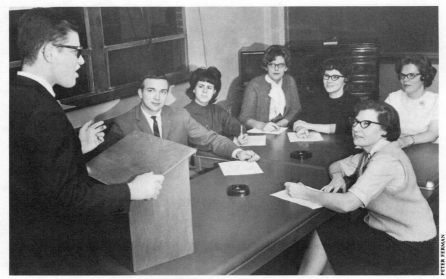

A deaf adult addresses a committee meeting.

6. *Another ear:* It is advisable for the deaf talker to develop a special relationship with a normally-hearing person or two who can act as a constructive and sympathetic critic of his speech. Care should be taken that the friend's judgment is not blunted by "getting used to" the speech. The other ear may, if desired, be a properly qualified professional who understands and is able to meet the distinctive speech needs of the adult deaf person.

7. *Public speaking:* It is encouraging that deaf persons are being called on to speak publicly. This requires suitable accommodation to public address systems. Among the sources of difficulty for the deaf speaker, as they may be for the hearing, are imperfections in the amplifying system, poor visibility of the face, and improper estimation of effects of distance from and angle to the microphone. These difficulties are best overcome by the use of a lavaliere microphone. We recommend testing a particular system before a speech is given, and enlisting the assistance of a hearing person and a monitor in the back of the room during the speech.

REVIEWING RESULTS

As we have seen, assessment of speech should determine aptitude for learning it, influence decisions about choice of method, and analyze deviations. In Chapter V we have discussed assessment of aptitude for learning speech as judged by specific criteria relating to the child's progress, special problems,

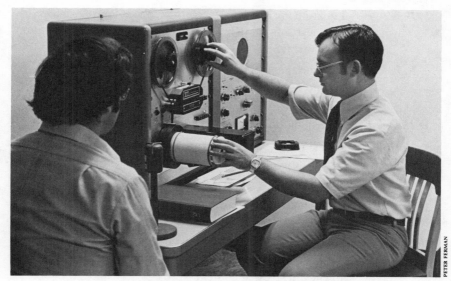

Spectrographic analysis to study speech production.

and the maintenance of a favorable environment. The assessment of aptitude leads to decisions about choice of emphasis on a particular "method." Analysis for deviations, sometimes referred to as "diagnosis," should be based on the deviations discussed in Chapter IV and in this chapter.

An interesting point of departure that may yield a measure of the quality of speech expressible as a numerical figure has been suggested by Monsen (163), who has been investigating speech of deaf children at Central Institute for the Deaf. Using spectrographic analysis, he compared six individual but overlapping aspects of speech of normal and deaf talkers. The first three of these indices deal primarily with segmental phonemic characteristics and the last three with suprasegmental or prosodic features. Preliminary investigations have included as speech samples reading of short lists of words in isolation, reading of a short paragraph or several individual sentences, and the production of isolated elongated vowels. The aspects of speech under investigation follow:

1. Primarily Segmental Indices

a. Index of: Coordination of laryngeal and oral articulatory gestures; accuracy of articulatory movement; distinctiveness of phoneme images.

Substance: Measurement of the ratio of voice onset time of stressed syllable initial **p t k** to that of **b d g**.

b. Index of: Location of phoneme targets in phonological space; distinctness of phoneme images; accuracy of articulatory movement.

Substance: Measurement of the difference in frequency between the second formant of **ee** and **oo**; measurement of the difference in frequency between the first formant of **ee** and **a(r)**.

c. Index of: Coarticulation of phonemes; duration control.

Substance: Measurement of the average vowel duration difference between vowels followed by voiced consonants and vowels followed by voiceless consonants.

2. Suprasegmental (Prosodic) Indices

d. Index of: Pitch control.

Substance: Measurement of the average change in fundamental frequency in stressed content words.

e. Index of: Duration control.

Substance: Measurement of the ratio of the average duration of three word classes: (1) unstressed function words, (2) stressed content words, and (3) content words in pre-pausal position or with contrastive stress.

f. Index of: Intensity control.

Substance: Measurement of the dB ratio of stressed and unstressed syllables.

The extent to which any one of these measures or combinations of them correlate with intelligibility remains to be determined.

To review results it is important to stand back from day-to-day activities—in other words, to ask how well we are doing. The "we" refers to child and teacher. Since our aim is intelligible speech, the assessment should focus on intelligibility and the possibility of modifying the program of an individual child or even the program of a school. Furthermore, intelligibility, along with the talker's confidence and usage, form the basis for prediction of the effectiveness of a talker's speech in academic, social, and vocational situations.

Evaluations can be made periodically during the school career of a deaf child when he is exposed to formal training in speech by one method or another. Other long-range procedures could be designed to discover how intelligible the speech of deaf pupils continues to be after they have graduated from special schools or classes.

A child's improvement in speech intelligibility may be evaluated by periodic tests, but the available tests are not as objective or as valid as our corresponding tests of many other skills or of a child's mastery of subject matter. In one popular procedure a child reads a selection and auditors indicate the extent to which the selection has been understood. Or, carefully selected word samples are read and scored by the auditors. In a sense, the tests determine the extent to which the deviant talker imposes a loss of discrimination for speech on a normal listener. Although this may yield a limited but fairly reasonable appraisal of the mechanics of the child's speech, it does not simulate the pattern of usual oral intercourse which takes place without benefit of a printed or written visual aid. What is being evaluated is a form of **oral reading** and not speech in broad social terms. The translation of a child's *own* thoughts into intelligible speech is an ability neglected by this type of evaluation.

The use of memorized material without visual aid is subject to similar criticism since the thoughts expressed usually are not the child's own; or, if they are, they have been memorized. This furnishes the child an advantage which he does not have in a normal social situation. The interview, in which the child is stimulated to talk freely, may yield a fairly accurate appraisal of speech if it is conducted skillfully. Very often in an interview, however, the questions influence the message set of a listener; furthermore, the technique fails to appraise the child's ability to initiate speech. The use of speech recordings for periodic evaluation has considerable value. However, the limitations of printed or memorized selections and of the question-and-answer type of sample should be kept in mind. Of course, it would help to capture for study the casual conversation of children. We should be cautious about the inferences we make that relate tests of talker intelligibility to social usefulness of speech. The two are not always linearly related. Attitudes of talker and listener having to do with confidence, encouragement, frustration, motivation—all these play their role in the use a deaf person makes of his speech.

The outcomes of speech teaching which are most important in the long run are those that reveal the extent to which the benefits of a child's training in speech persist after he has left school. Unfortunately, we have no satisfactory evidence in this area, and the information that comes to us is frequently biased and invariably anecdotal. Good follow-up studies are needed.

Some final comments are in order. The central theme of our treatise has been to enhance the teacher's power of analysis of the task of teaching speech, out of which grow the practical procedures to develop, improve, and maintain the speech of deaf persons. We have organized what we believe to be knowledge pertinent to the task, some of it documented and some based on experience. Students of speech of deaf children have been greatly stimulated by the development of improved tools and methods for the investigation of speech as an acoustic event. We now have techniques for analyzing and synthesizing speech, for making it available for visible and tactual display, and for manipulating it by selective filtering, frequency transposition, and temporal expansion and compression. These should aid our analysis of the perceptual features of speech and guide us in its appropriate manipulation for the benefit of the speech development of our children whose range of perceptual cues of speech are severely limited. The design of hearing aids and their use in auditory training are likely to be influenced significantly by the knowledge we acquire about the perception of speech. Our understanding of the physiological mechanisms of speech should be enriched by the techniques of high-speed photography of the larynx during phonation and of X-ray views of the articulators in action. Helpful, too, is our study of speech that is deviant because of such structural pathologies as cleft palate, vocal nodules, absent or partially removed larynx, or deficient innervation of speech musculature as in cerebral palsy.

Nevertheless, knowledge—however well organized, documented, and mastered—is not likely to be the exclusive ingredient for success. What eludes precise specification is the relationship that a teacher develops between herself and a student. Does the student feel "bad" when he is corrected or does he feel that the correction is made by someone who cares for him and in whom he has confidence? Does the teacher sense that too frequent interruption of an enthusiastic flow of language and thought in order to correct speech may degrade motivation for oral expression and, in the process, contribute to an abrasive teacher-student relationship? Does the worthwhileness of the effort to achieve spoken language permeate the atmosphere of the classroom? Does the lack of instant success lead to despair, resignation, or challenge? The answers to these and similar questions constitute the ingredient frequently referred to as "artistry" which, coupled with a sound scientific and empirical base, is the hallmark of the great teacher. In the face of the discouraging, the puzzling, the difficult, the unknown, and the deviant, she seeks *and is likely to find* a way to constructive action.

Appendix

Scales of Early Communication Skills for Hearing Impaired Children

Jean S. Moog and Ann V. Geers
Central Institute for the Deaf

The Scales of Early Communication Skills for Hearing Impaired Children are designed to evaluate speech and language development of children between the ages of 2 and 8 years. The instrument is divided into four scales: Receptive Language Skills, Expressive Language Skills, Non-Verbal Receptive Skills, and Non-Verbal Expressive Skills.

The Scales of Early Communication Skills for Hearing Impaired Children are completed by the child's teacher. Most other measures of language development are made by parent interview or by observation of the child in a test situation. Since communication behaviors are easily influenced by the subtleties of a situation, a very young child may not exhibit his best performance in a test situation. Therefore it is important that the child be evaluated by someone who knows him well and can observe his communication behavior in a variety of situations. A person who knows how to evaluate language is better able to make accurate ratings than an untrained person such as a parent. Therefore the child's teacher is the best choice as evaluator because she knows the child and knows how to rate language ability.

The rating form for the Scales of Early Communication Skills does not provide sufficient information for administering the scales. The items as listed do not fully describe the skill being rated, but rather serve as summary statements to cue the experienced rater. A manual which accompanies the Scales of Early Communication Skills thoroughly describes each item in terms of

197

the rationale for inclusion, criteria necessary for achieving a particular rating, and examples of behaviors which demonstrate the particular skill being rated. The authors consider the manual essential for appropriate use of the scales. Copies of the manual may be obtained by writing Central Institute for the Deaf, 818 South Euclid, St. Louis, Missouri 63110, Attention: Mr. Gjerdingen.

RATING FORM

SCALES OF EARLY COMMUNICATION SKILLS FOR HEARING IMPAIRED CHILDREN □□

□□□□□□□□

Name _____

Date _____ Child's Age _____

□□ □ □□

□ □□

RECEPTIVE LANGUAGE SKILLS

I.   DEMONSTRATES AWARENESS THAT THE MOUTH AND/ OR VOICE CONVEY INFORMATION.

22 □

_____ A. Responds to a verbal stimulus.

_____ B. Watches and/or listens to the speaker sponta-   □ neously.

II. DEMONSTRATES COMPREHENSION OF A FEW WORDS OR EXPRESSIONS.

24 □

_____ A. Identifies at least one word or expression from a   □ choice of two or three.

_____ B. Demonstrates comprehension of at least one word or   □ expression when situational cues are minimal and no gestures are used.

III. DEMONSTRATES THE ABILITY TO LEARN NEW WORDS.

26 □

_____ A. Identifies four or more words or expressions from a   □ choice of four or more.

_____ B. Demonstrates comprehension of four or more words,   □ phrases, or sentences when situational cues are minimal and no gestures are used.

IV. DEMONSTRATES THE ABILITY TO ACQUIRE NEW COM-
PREHENSION VOCABULARY IN PHRASES AND SEN-
TENCES.

28
_____ A. Learns new words in phrases and sentences after only □
a few exposures.

_____ B. Demonstrates ability to learn new words, phrases, □
and sentences outside the classroom.

V. DEMONSTRATES COMPREHENSION OF SUCCESSIVE
PHRASES AND SENTENCES.

30
_____ A. Demonstrates comprehension of the essential mean- □
ing of stories or related sentences about a particular
topic.

_____ B. Engages in conversation about a particular topic. □

EXPRESSIVE LANGUAGE SKILLS

I. DEMONSTRATES AWARENESS THAT VOCALIZATIONS
ARE USED TO COMMUNICATE.

32
_____ A. Vocalizes when expected to imitate speech. □

_____ B. Vocalizes spontaneously while looking at another □
person or to get someone's attention.

II. DEMONSTRATES THE ABILITY TO USE A FEW SYL-
LABLES, WORDS, OR EXPRESSIONS.

34
_____ A. Imitates at least one phoneme, syllable, or word. □

_____ B. Uses at least one syllable, word, or expression con- □
sistently and meaningfully.

III. DEMONSTRATES THE ABILITY TO LEARN NEW EX-
PRESSIVE VOCABULARY.

36
_____ A. Imitates at least four different syllables, words, or □
expressions.

_____ B. Uses at least four different words or expressions to □
communicate.

IV. DEMONSTRATES THE ABILITY TO ACQUIRE NEW EX-PRESSIVE VOCABULARY FAIRLY READILY.

38 ☐

_____ A. Imitates a large number of words or expressions af-ter only one or two presentations.

_____ B. Uses a variety of one-word utterances or expressions ☐ in spontaneous speech.

V. DEMONSTRATES THE ABILITY TO JOIN TWO OR THREE WORDS TOGETHER.

40 ☐

_____ A. Imitates at least two words of a phrase or recalls at least two words of a practiced sentence pattern.

_____ B. Joins at least two words in spontaneous speech. ☐

VI. DEMONSTRATES THE ABILITY TO USE VERBS IN TWO- TO THREE-WORD PHRASES OR SENTENCES.

42 ☐

_____ A. Imitates the verb and at least one other word of a phrase or recalls the verb and at least one other word of a practiced sentence pattern.

_____ B. Joins at least two words (one of which is a verb) in ☐ spontaneous speech.

VII. DEMONSTRATES THE ABILITY TO USE PHRASES OF FOUR OR MORE WORDS.

44 ☐

_____ A. Imitates at least four words of a phrase or recalls at least four words of a practiced sentence pattern.

_____ B. Uses phrases of four or more words in spontaneous ☐ speech.

VIII. DEMONSTRATES THE ABILITY TO USE SENTENCES OF SIX OR MORE WORDS CONTAINING MORE THAN ONE TYPE OF MODIFYING WORD OR PHRASE.

46 ☐

_____ A. Imitates or recalls practiced sentences containing more than one type of modifying word or phrase.

_____ B. Uses sentences containing more than one type of ☐ modifying word or phrase in spontaneous speech.

IX. DEMONSTRATES THE ABILITY TO USE SENTENCES OF EIGHT OR MORE WORDS CONTAINING MORE THAN ONE VERB FORM.

48 ☐

_____ A. Imitates or recalls practiced sentences containing more than one verb form.

_____ B. Uses sentences containing more than one verb form in spontaneous speech. ☐

NON-VERBAL RECEPTIVE SKILLS

50 ☐

_____ I. DEMONSTRATES THE ABILITY TO RESPOND APPROPRIATELY TO A SIMPLE GESTURE.

51 ☐

_____ II. DEMONSTRATES THE ABILITY TO RESPOND TO SUBTLE OR ELABORATE GESTURES WHEN THE SITUATION DOES NOT MAKE THE MEANING OBVIOUS.

52 ☐

_____ III. MAKES MAXIMUM USE OF WHATEVER CUES ARE AVAILABLE TO SUPPLEMENT THE WORDS HE KNOWS.

NON-VERBAL EXPRESSIVE SKILLS

53 ☐

_____ I. COMMUNICATES BY USING SIMPLE GESTURES.

54 ☐

_____ II. COMMUNICATES BY USING ELABORATE GESTURES.

55 ☐

_____ III. COMMUNICATES BY USING GESTURES OR PANTOMIME TO EXPRESS MORE THAN ONE IDEA OR RELATE SEQUENTIAL EVENTS.

56 ☐☐

Evaluated by _____

Bibliography and Suggested Readings

This bibliography is organized into three main sections to aid reader selection. They are: A. Methods, Techniques, and Related Comments; B. Relevant Research and Comments; and C. More Research and General Background. While reasonable reservations might be made about the classification of a number of entries in particular sections, we consider the organization to be fundamentally useful. We have chosen a representative sample of entries for annotation to illustrate the kinds of helpful material available in the professional and scientific literature.

SECTION A.
METHODS, TECHNIQUES, and RELATED COMMENTS

1. Alcorn, S. K. The Tadoma method. *The Volta Review,* 1932, **34,** 195–198.
2. Alcorn, S. K. Speech development through vibration. *The Volta Review*, 1938, **40,** 633–637.
3. Alcorn, S. K. Development of Speech by the Tadoma method. In *Report of Proceedings of the 32nd Meeting of the Convention of American Instructors of the Deaf, 1941.* Washington, D. C.: U. S. Government Printing Office, 1942, 241–243.

   These three articles (also see Gruver) are brief descriptions, supplementing each other, of the Tadoma method, an approach to teaching speech in which much importance is given to the pupil's placing his hand on the teacher's face to feel vibrations and muscle movement.

4. Angelocci, A. A. Some observations on the speech of the deaf. *The Volta Review,* 1962, **74,** 403–405.

5. Avery, C. B. Orthographic systems used in education of the deaf. *The Volta Review,* 1967, **69,** 208–210.

6. Avondino, J. The Babbling method. *The Volta Review,* 1918, **20,** 667–671, 767–771; 1919, **21,** 67–71, 142–145, 224–228, 273–282.
   The rationale and the procedures of a technique for developing, perfecting, and maintaining speech by drilling on nonsense syllables. A graded series of drill exercises, in which phonemes occur in a wide variety of contexts, is presented. The exercises aim at leading gradually from elemental and easy syllables to complex and difficult combinations. Explanations and teaching suggestions accompany the exercises.

7. Beebe, H. H. *A guide to help the severely hard-of-hearing child.* Basel, Switzerland: S. Karger, 1953.
   One of the original books on the auditory approach. Available through the Alexander Graham Bell Association, Washington, D.C.

8. Bell, A. G. *The mechanism of speech.* New York: Funk and Wagnalls Company, 1907.
   Lectures to teachers by A. G. Bell. "When the lectures were originally delivered, the teachers present were encouraged to ask questions concerning difficulties experienced in imparting the power of articulate speech to deaf children. In this volume the questions and answers have been appended to the lectures, in the hope that the replies may be of assistance to other teachers engaged in this difficult and laborious work."

9. Boothroyd, A., Archambault, P., Adams, R. E., & Storm, R.D. Use of a computer-based system of speech training aids for deaf persons. *The Volta Review,* 1975, **77,** 178–193.

10. Calvert, D. R. Speech sound duration and the surd-sonant error. *The Volta Review,* 1962, **64,** 401–402.
    A short discussion of differences in the duration of segments of some of the consonants in the speech of deaf talkers compared with the speech of normally-hearing talkers.

11. Calvert, D. R. An approach to the study of deaf speech. *Report of Proceedings of the International Congress on Education of the Deaf and the 41st Meeting of the Convention of American Instructors of the Deaf, 1963.* Washington, D.C.: U.S. Government Printing Office, 1964, 242–245.

12. Clarke School for the Deaf. *Auditory training*. Special Study Institute, Curriculum Evaluation and Development Program, Auditory Training Handbook, Curriculum Series, Northampton, Massachusetts, 1971.

13. Clarke School for the Deaf. *Speech*. Special Study Institute, Curriculum Evaluation and Development Program, Speech Development, Curriculum Series, Northampton, Massachusetts, 1971.

14. Connor, L. E. (Ed.). *Speech for the deaf child: Knowledge and use*. Washington, D.C.: Alexander Graham Bell Association for the Deaf, 1971.
    A monograph addressed to teachers and allied workers interested in speech for the deaf. Includes sections on speech science, speech development and disorders, speech teaching, and organizational patterns.

15. Cornett, R. O. Oralism vs. manualism, the method explained, cued speech. *Hearing-Speech News,* 1967, **35,** 7–9.

16. Cornett, R. O. Cued speech. In *Report of Proceedings of the 43rd Meeting of the Convention of American Instructors of the Deaf, 1967*. Washington, D.C.: U.S. Government Printing Office, 1968, 112–113.
    Brief, very general descriptions of cued speech, a system of hand signals whose purpose is to make lipreading easier.

17. Cued Speech. *The Australian Teacher of the Deaf,* 1970, **11,** 153–165.
    Assessments of cued speech, by principals of schools for the deaf where it has been tried.

18. DiCarlo, L. S. Speech: Deed or dream. In L. S. DiCarlo (Ed.), *The deaf*. Englewood, N.J.: Prentice Hall, 1964. (Chapter 4, pp. 88–116.)

19. Doehring, D. G., & Ling, D. Programmed instruction of hearing-impaired children in the auditory discrimination of vowels. *Journal of Speech and Hearing Research,* 1971, **14,** 746–753.

20. Eilers, R. E., & Minifie, F. D. Fricative discrimination in early infancy. *Journal of Speech and Hearing Research,* 1975, **18,** 158–167.

21. Erber, N. P., & Greer, C. W. Communication strategies used by teachers at an oral school for the deaf. *The Volta Review,* 1973, **75,** 480–485.

22. Erber, N. P. Effects of angle, distance, and illumination on visual reception of speech by profoundly deaf children. *Journal of Speech and Hearing Research,* 1974, **17,** 99–112.

23. Erber, N. P., & Zeiser, M. L. Classroom observation under conditions

of simulated profound deafness. *The Volta Review,* 1974, **76,** 352–360.

24. Ewing A., & Ewing, E. C. *Teaching deaf children to talk.* Manchester, England: Manchester University Press, 1964.

25. Ewing, A. Speech—some teaching methodology. *Proceedings of the International Conference on Oral Education of the Deaf.* Washington, D.C.: The Alexander Graham Bell Association for the Deaf, 1967, 556–563.

26. Ewing, I. R., & Ewing, A. W. G. *Speech and the deaf child.* Washington, D.C.: The Alexander Graham Bell Association for the Deaf, 1954. The authors are strong proponents of oral communication. This book is a general presentation of their approach to teaching speech. Speech in their view is the capacity to understand the spoken word, to use it, and to take part in conversation. Includes sections on the history of the teaching of speech to the deaf, needs of the deaf child, and methods of developing speech.

27. Fairbanks, G. *Voice and articulation drillbook* (2nd ed.). New York: Harper and Brothers, Publishers, 1959. Drill materials and instructions for improving pronunciation, breathing, timing, loudness, pitch, intonation, voice quality, and general expressiveness. Not addressed specifically to the speech of the deaf. Contains suggestions on how to evaluate speech quality, and a section on articulation describes the common phonemes of English in terms of their place and manner of articulation and their spellings.

28. Fellendorf, G. (Ed.). *Proceedings of the International Conference on Oral Education of the Deaf.* (2 vols.) Washington, D.C.: The Alexander Graham Bell Association for the Deaf, 1967. Report in two volumes (2211 pages) of a conference observing the centennial of oral education of the deaf in the United States. Includes papers by world experts on identification of deafness, organization and administration of services, speech, auditory training, preparation of professional personnel, instruction in language, curriculum development, and educational trends. The following papers from these proceedings pertain to speech for hearing impaired children.

28.1 Numbers, M. E. A plea for better speech, **1,** 543–555.
28.2 Ewing, A. W. G. Speech—some teaching methodology, **1,** 556–563.

28.3   Calvert, D. R. A descriptive outline of the act of teaching speech, **1**, 581–598.

28.4   Thomasia, M. Speech, **1**, 599–613.

28.5   French, S. L. Implications of information theory for speech for the deaf, **1**, 614–628.

28.6   Nicholas, M. Speech methodology at St. Mary's School for the Deaf, **1**, 629–643.

28.7   Harrell, H. Speech: An integrated subject, **1**, 644–651.

28.8   Lorenz, M. L. A speech program for deaf children from ten to fifteen, **1**, 652–663.

28.9   Krijnen, A. Developing the voices of very young deaf children, **1**, 664–671.

28.10 Schmaehl, O. Speech education for mentally retarded deaf children, **1**, 672–679.

28.11 Rozanska, E. v. D. An approach to teaching speech to the deaf, **1**, 680–684.

28.12 Carr, J. The role of the teacher educator in improving speech for the deaf, **1**, 685–704.

28.13 Berg, F. S., & Fletcher, S. G. The hard-of-hearing child and educational audiology, **1**, 874–885.

28.14 Woodward, H. M. E. Intonation and the teaching of speech, **1**, 886–907.

29. Fry, D. B. The development of the phonological system in the normal and deaf child. In F. Smith & G. A. Miller (Eds.), *The genesis of language: A psycholinguistic approach.* Cambridge, Massachusetts: Massachusetts Institute of Technology Press, 1966, 187–206.

Presents a theory of how the normal child develops a phonological system, starting with the earliest exposure to speech and continuing to the child's establishment of a complete repertory of phonemes by about 7 years of age. Discusses the roles of auditory, tactile, and kinesthetic feedback; the contribution of babbling; and the importance of imitation and social reinforcement. Relates these ideas to the problem of speech acquisition by the deaf and outlines an approach for teaching deaf children based on auditory stimulation through speech, starting in infancy.

30. Gault, R. H. The use of the sense of touch in developing speech. *The Volta Review,* 1934, **36**, 82–83.

The author developed an aid which amplifies speech and presents it to the fingers through a vibrator. This article is a very brief sum-

mary of the aspects of speech which such a tactile device can help a
deaf person to perceive.

31. Goldstein, M. A. *The acoustic method for the training of the deaf and
hard-of-hearing child.* St. Louis, Missouri: The Laryngoscope
Press, 1939.
An early treatment of systematic auditory training. Author's
quote: "It is my sincere opinion that the principal reason for the
many unsuccessful attempts and indifferent results in the use of the
acoustic method are due to the desultory, aimless, and unsystemat-
ic form of procedure which has discouraged teacher and pupil alike
and which has given rise to so many misconceptions and misunder-
standings about this particular special pedagogy."

32. Griffiths, C. (Ed.) *International Conference on Auditory Techniques.*
Springfield, Illinois: Charles C Thomas, 1974.

33. Gruver, M. H. The Tadoma method. *The Volta Review,* 1955, **57,** 17–
19.
A description of the Tadoma method and a favorable report on its
use at a school for the deaf.

34. Guberina, P. Verbotonal method and its application to the rehabilitation of the deaf. *Report of Proceedings of the International Congress on Education of the Deaf and the 41st Meeting of the Convention of American Instructors of the Deaf, 1963.* Washington,
D.C., U.S. Government Printing Office, 1964, 279–293.
Largely devoted to the presentation of theoretical ideas about
speech perception which provide the author's rationale for his Verbotonal Method.

35. Haycock, G. S. *The teaching of speech.* Washington, D.C.: The Alexander Graham Bell Association for the Deaf, 1942.
First published in 1933 and repeatedly reprinted but not substantially revised, this book continues to be a basic reference for
teachers of speech to the deaf, despite its predating the widespread
use of electronic hearing aids. Contains systematic sets of procedures for teaching speech to deaf children. It emphasizes that
"speech is movement" and outlines approaches for developing natural speech, at the same time not ignoring the need—sooner or later—for specific articulation work. To this end, each English sound
is described, and practical advice is given on how to elicit it, drill
on it, and correct it if it is faulty.

36. Hirsh, I. J. Communication for the deaf. *Report of Proceedings of the International Congress on Education of the Deaf and the 41st Meeting of the Convention of American Instructors of the Deaf, 1963.* Washington, D.C.: U.S. Government Printing Office, 1964, 164–183.

   A description in broad strokes—based on phonetics, psycho-acoustics, and psychology—of what the task of teaching speech to the hearing handicapped consists of. Various definitions of deafness are considered, and the difficulties of using audiograms to describe and classify hearing impaired persons are explained. Examines some of the relations between different types of hearing losses and the acoustic properties of speech, discussing the nature of the acoustic information in speech which may be available—or may be made available—to the hearing impaired. Provides insight into the rationale of various approaches toward teaching speech to the deaf—for example, approaches which stress auditory training, or rhythm, or frequency shifting hearing aids, etc.

37. Hirsh, I. J. Teaching the deaf child to speak. In F. Smith & G. A. Miller (Eds.), *The genesis of language: A psycholinguistic approach.* Cambridge, Massachusetts: The Massachusetts Institute of Technology Press, 1966, 207–216.

38. Holbrook, A. Procedures for conditioning deaf infants with speech teaching machines. (Paper presented at Norrkoping, Sweden, for the European Association for Special Education, July, 1971; and at the World Federation of the Deaf, Paris, France, August 1971.)

39. Holbrook, A., & Crawford, G. H. Modification of speech behavior in the speech of the deaf—hypernasality. (Excerpts from a paper presented to the Conference of Executives of American Schools for the Deaf, and included in its proceedings. St. Augustine, Florida, April 1970.)

40. Holbrook, A., & Crawford, G. H. Modifications of vocal frequency and intensity in the speech of the deaf. *The Volta Review*, 1970, **72,** 492–297.

   Describes an operant conditioning apparatus (FLORIDA) using a timer and on-off lights to signal whether speech is within acceptable pitch and intensity ranges. Procedures for using it to modify the speech of deaf persons are outlined.

41. Hudgins, C. V. A comparative study of the speech coordinations of deaf and normal subjects. *Journal of Genetic Psychology*, 1934, **44**, 1–48.

   The author measured and compared the air pressures and muscle movements in the speech breathing of hearing impaired and normally-hearing children. The report is rich in background information and clear explanations about speech breathing, syllabification, accent grouping, phrasing, the releasing and arresting functions of consonants, breathiness, nasality, and voice-unvoiced consonant contrasts. Sheds light on a wide range of defects in the speech of deaf children which have little to do with the accuracy of individual element articulation but rather are related to poor coordination of the total speech producing system.

42. Hudgins, C. V., & Numbers, F. C. An investigation of intelligibility of speech of the deaf. *Genetic Psychology Monographs*, 1942, **25**, 289–392.

   Analysis of the speech of 192 pupils in two schools for the deaf, with two main purposes: to identify speech errors, classify them, and determine their frequency of occurrence; and to determine the relative effects of each type of error on speech intelligibility. Two major classes of errors were considered: errors of articulation and errors of rhythm. Articulation errors were found to fall into seven categories for consonants and five categories for vowels. In addition to examining the importance of each category of error with reference to intelligibility, the authors correlate the various kinds of errors with degree of hearing loss and age of speakers. The authors also rank the phonemes of English according to their difficulty as determined by frequency of error in the speech of the deaf. This monograph continues the discussion of many of the ideas of Hudgins, particularly those concerning speech breathing, releasing and arresting functions of consonants, and the concept that unintelligibility results from incoordination of the total speech system. Argues strongly against basing the teaching of speech on the teaching of individual element articulation.

43. Hudgins, C. V. Speech intelligibility tests: A practical program. *The Volta Review*, 1943, **45**, 52–54.

   A description of a Clarke School for the Deaf speech intelligibility testing program based on the intelligibility of whole sentences.

44. Hudgins, C. V. Speech breathing and intelligibility. *The Volta Review,* 1946, **48,** 642–644.

Discusses the importance of controlling breath to form the syllable groupings and rhythms of normal-sounding speech. Types of speech rhythm defects related to improper breath control are listed, and their destructive effect on intelligibility is stressed. A type of teaching which fosters improper breath control, and is therefore to be avoided, is described; and a teaching approach which would help develop proper speech breathing is outlined.

45. Hudgins, C. V. A method of appraising the speech of the deaf. *The Volta Review,* 1949, **51,** 597–601, 638.

Describes a test in which deaf children are scored on the intelligibility of their pronunciation of lists of PBF (Phonetically Balanced Familiar) words. The method of testing is an application of the Bell Telephone Laboratories "Articulation Testing Method" commonly used to test speech intelligibility but not necessarily involving deaf speakers. The selection and training of judges is discussed, and the effects on their judgments of experience gained during the testing program are considered. A graph is presented showing a relationship which the author found between intelligibility scores on word list tests and on whole sentence tests; the possibility of predicting the score on the one kind of test from the score of the other kind is indicated.

46. Jeffers, J. Formants and the auditory training of deaf children. *The Volta Review,* 1966, **68,** 418–423, 449.

A broad and simplified explanation of vowel formants. Frequencies of the second formants of the English vowels and diphthongs are listed for men, women, and children. Presents a simplified idea of the frequency capabilities required of both hearing aids and listeners in order for any particular vowel or diphthong to be reproduced and perceived fairly completely.

47. Joiner, E. Our speech teaching heritage. *The Volta Review,* 1948, **50,** 417–422.

Contains practical information about teaching speech from the point of view of an experienced teacher of the deaf whose approach is strongly analytical, stressing conscious, precise control of the articulators.

48. John Tracy Clinic. *Teaching speech to the profoundly deaf. Study guide for the film series.* Los Angeles, California, The John Tracy Clinic, 1970.

49. Kelly, J. C. *Clinician's handbook for auditory training* (2nd Ed.). Washington, D.C.: The Alexander Graham Bell Association for the Deaf, 1973.

   A workbook of exercise material for use with adults and older children in conjunction with other habilitation materials.

50. Laurentine, M. The speech program at St. Joseph Institute for the Deaf. *The Volta Review,* 1964, 66, 459–463.

51. Leshin, G. (Ed.), Pearce, M. F., & Funderburg, R. S. *Speech for the hearing impaired child.* Tucson, Arizona: University of Arizona, Department of Special Education, College of Education, 1974.

   Suggests specific techniques.

52. Levitt, H., & Nye, P. W. (Eds.) *Proceedings of the Conference on Sensory Training Aids for the Hearing Impaired.* Washington, D.C., 1971.

   A conference of engineers, speech scientists, electroacousticians, psychoacousticians, and educators of the deaf.

53. Ling, D. An auditory approach to the education of deaf children. *Audecibel,* 1964, 13, 96–101.

   A unisensory approach.

54. Lyon, E. *The Lyon phonetic manual.* Rochester, New York: American Association To Promote the Teaching of Speech to the Deaf, Circulation of Information #2, 1891.

55. Magner, M. E. Beginning speech for young deaf children. *The Volta Review,* 1953, 55, 20–23.

56. Mártony, J. Visual aids for speech correction. In G. Fant (Ed.), *Proceedings of the International Symposium on Speech Communication Ability and Profound Deafness, Stockholm, Sweden, 1970.* Washington, D.C.: The Alexander Graham Bell Association for the Deaf, 1972.

57. McGinnis, M. A. *Aphasic children: Identification and education by the Association method.* Washington, D.C.: The Alexander Graham Bell Association for the Deaf, 1963.

   Detailed exposition of the principles and techniques of what in the present book we have called the Association Phoneme Unit method.

58. Moog, J. S. Approaches to teaching pre-primary hearing impaired children. *Bulletin: American Organization for the Education of the Hearing Impaired,* 1973, 1(3), 52–59.

59. Moores, D. F. Neo-oralism and the education of the deaf. *Exceptional Children*, 1972, **38**, 377–384.

    Cites rejection of teaching speech by simple sound/letter relations even with fingerspelling. Mentions briefly a "concentric" method of teaching speech which concentrates initially on a limited number of sounds for 42 letters.

60. New, M. C. Speech for the young deaf child. *The Volta Review*, 1940, **42**, 592–599.

    Describes the "natural" approach to teaching speech used at the Lexington School. Presents the year-by-year objectives and some of the teaching procedures of a curriculum which from the very beginning uses whole words and flowing language to stimulate nursery-age children to communicate orally with natural rhythm and natural language. Precise articulation is developed through perfecting the pronunciation of whole words and phrases, and only later through conscious control of individual elements. Contrasts this with programs which concentrate first on perfecting the speech of individual elements.

61. New, M. Color in speech teaching. *The Volta Review*, 1942, **44**, 133–138, 199–203.

62. Numbers, M. E. The place of elements in speech development. *The Volta Review*, 1942, **44**, 261–265.

    Argues strongly against the teaching of isolated, discrete articulation elements. Favors basing the teaching of speech on the teaching of whole syllables, with the elements taught as movements within a specific, indivisible syllable or word context. Discusses speech breathing and rhythm, and explains the releasing and arresting functions of consonants.

63. Pickett, J. M. (Ed.) Proceedings of the Conference on Speech-Analyzing Aids for the Deaf. Hearing and Speech Center, Gallaudet College, Washington, D.C., 1967. *American Annals of the Deaf*, 1968, **113**(2), 116–330.

    This issue is devoted to the proceedings of a 1967 conference on speech-analyzing aids for the deaf. A substantial portion of the issue is concerned with the use of instruments to transmit information about speech to the hearing impaired and aimed at the development and improvement of their speech. The following papers may be of particular interest to teachers of the deaf:

63.1 Pickett, J. M. Sound patterns of speech: An introductory sketch, 120–126.
This paper describes and classifies the phonemes of English in terms of some of their acoustical features.

63.2 Liberman, A. M., Cooper, F. S.,Shankweiler, D. P., & Studdert-Kennedy, M. Why are speech spectrograms hard to read?, 127–133.
A discussion of the major theoretical difficulty in displaying speech visually. The paper emphasizes the complexities of the interrelationships of phonemes with their contexts.

63.3 Stewart, R. B. By ear alone, 147–155.
Points out some of the difficulties a listener encounters in analyzing and transcribing the speech of deaf children. Discusses some of the characteristics of speech which must be taken into account in making judgments about speech quality.

63.4 Børrild, K. Experience with the design and use of technical aids for the training of deaf and hard of hearing children, 168–177.
Briefly describes and comments on the usefulness of speech training devices using visual displays which have been tried out at a school for the deaf in Denmark. These include "S" indicators and indicators of pitch, loudness, and spectrum.

63.5 Risberg, A. Visual aids for speech correction, 178–194.
Discusses theoretical reasons why visual display devices should be useful for teaching speech. Describes the following instruments which have been used in his laboratory: a spectrum indicator, a fricative indicator, an "S" indicator, an intonation indicator, a rhythm indicator, and a nasalization indicator. An experiment to test the teaching value of an "S" indicator is reported.

63.6 Mártony, J. On the correction of the voice pitch level for severely hard of hearing subjects, 195–202.
Discusses the association of involuntary pitch changes with particular phonemes and the use of a visual pitch indicator by deaf children to help them improve their voices.

63.7 Stark, R. E., Cullen J. K. Jr., & Chase, R. Preliminary work with the new Bell Telephone visible speech translator, 205–214.
Summarizes the results of use of "visible speech" to modify abnormally high pitch, incorrect, tuning, excessive nasaliza-

tion, and articulation of hearing impaired children and adults. Suggestions for teachers who might use a visible speech device are offered.

63.8 Pronovost, W., Yenkin, L., & Anderson, D. C. The voice visualizer, 230–238.

63.9 Phillips, N. D., Remillard, W., & Bass, S. Teaching of intonation to the deaf by visual pattern matching, 239–245.

63.10 Cohen, M. L. The ADL sustained phoneme analyzer, 247–252.

63.11 Pickett, J. M., & Constam, A. A visual speech trainer with simplified indication of vowel spectrum, 253–258.

63.12 Ling, D. Three experiments on frequency transposition, 283–294.
Reports experiments designed to test the value of hearing aids which transpose speech into the low frequencies available to many deaf persons.

63.13 Guttman, N., & Nelson, R. An instrument that creates some artificial speech spectra for the severely hard of hearing, 295–302.
The authors report on a hearing aid which adds low frequency energy to phonemes which might otherwise be inaudible because they normally consist mostly of high frequencies.

63.14 Kringelbotn, M. Experiments with some visual and vibrotactile aids for the deaf, 311–317.

64. Pollack, D. *Educational audiology for the limited hearing infant.* Springfield, Illinois: Charles C Thomas, 1970.
The principles and procedures of acoupedics, a comprehensive program of auditory training for teachers, clinicians, and parents.

65. Poulos, T. H. Improving the intelligibility of deaf children's speech. *The Volta Review,* 1952, **54,** 265–267.

66. Poulos, T. H. A speech improvement program in a large residential school for the deaf. *The Volta Review,* 1962, **64,** 405–408.

67. Pugh, B. Clarifying speech problems for the deaf. *The Volta Review,* 1963, **65,** 15–21.

68. Rockey, D. *Phonetic lexicon.* New York: Heyden and Son, Ltd., 1973.
A compilation of monosyllabic and some disyllabic words arranged according to their phonetic structure. A good source for drill and test material.

69. Ronnei, E. C., & Porter, J. *Tim and his hearing aid* (Rev. ed.). Washington, D.C.: The Alexander Graham Bell Association for the Deaf, 1965. (Spanish edition also available.)
A young boy learns to use a hearing aid.

70. Round Hill Round Table. In defense of the Northampton Charts. *The Volta Review,* 1942, **44,** 487.

71. Silverman, S. R. Teaching speech to the deaf: The issues. *The Volta Review,* 1954, **56,** 385–389, 417.
This paper summarizes and explains the issues in some important areas of disagreement among those who believe in teaching speech to the deaf. The areas of disagreement which are discussed are: Fundamental attitudes toward speech (For everyday communication? As a second language? . . .); Sensory approaches (Visual? Auditory? . . . One? Many? . . .); Orthography systems (Northampton? IPA? . . .); Basic units of speech (Elements? Syllables? Words? . . .); Evaluation of teaching (By oral reading? In real-life situations? . . .).

72. Simmons, A. A. Teaching aural language. *The Volta Review,* 1968, **70,** 26–30.
Stresses that in the education of young deaf children speech and language must not be separated from each other. What needs to be taught initially is oral-aural communication, not precise speech and precise language. Urges teachers to use multi-word phrases, not single words. Emphasizes the information-carrying significance of prosody and maintains that prosody is the first aspect of language to develop in hearing children and should be the first aspect developed in deaf children.

73. Simmons-Martin, A. The oral/aural procedure: Theoretical basis and rationale. *The Volta Review,* 1972, **74,** 541–551.

74. Stark, R. E. Teaching /ba/ and /pa/ to deaf children using real-time spectral displays. *Language and Speech,* 1972, **15,** 14–29.

75. Stetson, R. H. Contributions of teachers of the deaf to the science of phonetics. *The Volta Review,* 1943, **45,** 19–20; 54–56.
A historical note about some of the contributions which teachers of the deaf have made to the sciences of speech and hearing since Melville Bell produced his system of Visible Speech in 1867. Focuses on the ideas of those who emphasized that the dynamic nature of speech makes the syllable rather than the single element the

more useful unit on which to base the teaching of speech to deaf persons.

76. Stoner, M. The development of early speech with emphasis on the synthetic method. *The Volta Review*, 1955, **57**, 15–17.

77. Sweet, M. E. The association method for aphasics: Its application to the deaf. *The Volta Review*, 1955, **57**, 13–15.

78. Utley, J. *What's its name?* Urbana, Illinois: The University of Illinois Press, 1950.
A workbook designed for parents and teachers of preschool and primary age hearing impaired children. Auditory training album. Records to accompany *What's Its Name?*

79. van Uden, A. Instructing prelingually deaf children by the rhythms of bodily movements and of sounds, by oral mime and general bodily expression: its possibilities and difficulties. In *Report of Proceedings of the International Congress on Education of the Deaf and the 41st Meeting of the Convention of American Instructors of the Deaf, 1963.* Washington, D.C.: U.S. Government Printing Office, 1964, 852–873.

80. van Uden, A. New realizations in the light of the pure oral method. *The Volta Review*, 1970, **72**, 524–536.
Discusses some of the major points of the "Maternal Reflective Method" which is used to teach speech and language at Sint-Michielsgestel School for the Deaf in the Netherlands. Among the features of the program are: the goal is oral conversation, starting in childhood; all sensory channels are used; teaching is through conversations in which the teacher corrects and expands the children's own utterances; diaries of conversations are kept; great attention is paid to developing natural intonation and speech rhythm, especially accent groupings, based on the rationale that a feel for natural speech rhythm will help constrain a child into using correct language.

81. van Uden, A. *Dove Kinderen leren spreken (How children learn to speak).* Rotterdam, Holland: Universitaire Pers Rotterdam, 1974. (Summary in English.)

82. Vivian, R. M. The Tadoma method: A tactual approach to speech and speech reading. *The Volta Review*, 1966, **68**, 733–737.
A teacher at Perkins School for the Blind tells how the Tadoma method is used with deaf-blind children. Describes commonly used

positions of the hands on the face. Offers suggestions about stimulating awareness of vibration and developing tactual sensitivity
and tactual skills. Lists some exercises to build ability to imitate
the muscular movement of others. Briefly discusses some procedures for teaching speechreading and speech production.

83. Vorce, E. *Teaching speech to deaf children.* (The Lexington School for
the Deaf, Education Series, Book IX.) Washington, D.C.: The Alexander Graham Bell Association for the Deaf, 1974.
Organization and methods of the speech program at Lexington
School for the Deaf, New York.

84. Walter, B. Dynamic and formal elements in the teaching of spoken language to deaf children. In A. Ewing (Ed.), *The modern educational
treatment of deafness.* Manchester, England: Manchester University Press, 1960, 45/1–45/6.

85. Watson, T. J. Auditory training and the development of speech and language in children with defective hearing. *Acta Oto-Laryngologica,*
1951, **40,** 95–103.
Directed to participants in an audiology course, most of whom
were otologists and audiologists. The auditory training program to
which the author devotes most of his discussion is aimed at training profoundly deaf children to use their residual hearing to master
the prosodic features of speech and as an adjunct to lipreading.
Broad goals and activities for nursery, primary, and post-primary
programs are outlined.

86. Wedenberg, E. Auditory training of severely hard of hearing preschool
children. *Acta Oto-Laryngologica,* 1954, Supplement 110.

87. Whetnall, E., & Fry, D. B. *The deaf child.* London, England: William
Heinemann, 1964.
An exposition of the development of communication in deaf chil-
dren emphasizing an early auditory approach.

88. Whetnall, E., & Fry, D. B. *Learning to hear.* London, England: William
Heinemann, 1970. Washington, D.C.: R. B. Niven, Ed.

89. Whitehurst, M. W. *Auditory training for children.* (Rev. ed.) Armonk,
New York: Hearing Rehabilitation Co., 1966.
Graded lessons from very simple to difficult.

90. Yale, C. A. Dr. Bell's early experiments in giving speech to the deaf. *The
Volta Review,* 1927, **29,** 293–295.
Describes an experiment that Alexander Graham Bell conducted
at the Clarke School for the Deaf in the belief that knowledge of

the articulation positions of individual speech elements would result in better speech. The experiment involved vocal gymnastics and voiceless practicing of the mechanical actions of speech, without actually speaking. Tells of Bell's training a very deaf girl to sound the eight notes of the musical scale and to sing a tune.

91. Yale, C. A. *Formation and development of elementary English sounds.* Northampton, Massachusetts: Metcalf, 1938.

The Northampton Charts and their rationale. An accompanying explication of each sound on the charts describes the production of the sound and gives suggestions on how to elicit it from a deaf child.

92. Zaliouk, A. A visual-tactile system of phonetical symbolization. *Journal of Speech and Hearing Disorders,* 1954, **19**, 190–207.

Concerned with labeling each phoneme, with both pictures and hand cues, to show the articulator positions and movements for the phoneme and also to indicate the tactile information which production of the phoneme generates. Lists finger and hand placements for doing this. Presents a system for diagramming phonemes, and offers a phonetic alphabet in which the symbols are pictographs of the articulators and also suggest tactile information.

SECTION B.
RELEVANT RESEARCH AND COMMENTS

93. Becking, A. G. T. Perception of airborne sound in the thorax of deaf children. In *Proceedings of the International Course in Paedo-audiology,* Groningen, Verenigde Drukkerijen Hoitsema, N. V., 1953, 88–97.

94. Beckwith, L. Relationships between infants' vocalizations and their mothers' behaviors. *Merrill Palmer Quarterly,* 1971, **17**, 211–216.

95. Bishop, M. E., Ringel, R. L., & House, A. S. Orosensory perception, speech production, and deafness. *Journal of Speech and Hearing Research,* 1973, **16**, 257–266.

96. Black, J. W. Experimental phonetics: What experimental phonetics has to offer the teacher of the deaf. *The Volta Review,* 1960, **62**, 313–315.

97. Blanton, R. L., Nunnally, J. C., & Odom, P. B. Graphemic, phonetic, and associative factors in the verbal behavior of deaf and hearing

subjects. *Journal of Speech and Hearing Research,* 1967, **10,** 225–231.

98. Blasdell, R., & Jensen, P. Stress and word position as determinants of imitation in first-language learners. *Journal of Speech and Hearing Research,* 1970, **13,** 193-202.

99. Boothroyd, A. Some experiments on the control of voice in the profoundly deaf using a pitch extractor and storage oscilloscope display. In C. P. Smith (Ed.), *Conference on Speech Communication and Processing.* Air Force Cambridge Research Laboratories, Cambridge, Massachusetts, AFCRL-72-0120, Special Report No. 131, 1972.

100. Brannon, J. B., Jr. Visual feedback of glossal motions and its influence on the speech of deaf children. Doctoral dissertation, Northwestern University, 1964.

101. Brannon, J. B., Jr. The speech production and spoken language of the deaf. *Language and Speech,* 1966, **9,** 127–135.
    A rapid survey of the speech and language defects of deaf persons.

102. *California state master plan for education of the deaf,* 1970. Sacramento, California: California Department of Education, 1970.

103. Calvert, D. R. Some acoustic characteristics of the speech of profoundly deaf individuals. Doctoral dissertation, Stanford University, 1961.

104. Calvert, D. R. Deaf voice quality: A preliminary investigation. *The Volta Review,* 1962, **64,** 402–403.
    A brief summary of research which indicates that "deaf voice" is not simply a matter of unnatural fundamental frequency and unusual harmonics.

105. Carr, J. Early speech development of deaf children. *Report of Proceedings of the International Congress on Education of the Deaf and the 41st Meeting of the Convention of American Instructors of the Deaf, 1963.* Washington, D.C.: U.S. Government Printing Office, 1964, 261–267.

106. Chen, M. Vowel length variation as a function of the voicing of the consonant environment. *Phonetics,* 1970, **22,** 129–159.

107. Cohen, M. L. The ADL sustained phoneme analyzer. *American Annals of the Deaf,* 1968, **113,** 247–252.

108. Colton, R. H., & Cooker, H. S. Perceived nasality in the speech of the deaf. *Journal of Speech and Hearing Research,* 1968, **11,** 553–559.
    Concludes that much of the perceived nasality in the speech of deaf persons may be a natural consequence of unnaturally slow speaking tempo.

109. Conrad, R. Short-term memory processes in the deaf. *British Journal of Psychology,* 1970, **61,** 179–195.
110. Conrad, R. Short-term memory in the deaf: A test for speech coding. *British Journal of Psychology,* 1972, **63,** 173–180.
111. Conrad, R. Some correlates of speech coding in the short-term memory of the deaf. *Journal of Speech and Hearing Research,* 1973, **16,** 375–384.
112. Davis, H., & Silverman, S. R. (Eds.) *Hearing and deafness* (3rd ed.). New York: Holt, Rinehart, and Winston, 1970.
    A comprehensive introductory text on audiology. Of particular interest to teachers of speech are chapters on acoustics and psychoacoustics, auditory tests, hearing aids, auditory training, speech development and conservation, and deaf children.
113. Denes, P. B. Speech science and the deaf. *The Volta Review,* 1968, **70,** 603–607.
    Describes the thus far insoluble problems which scientists have encountered with speech aids which transform speech into light patterns.
114. Dickson, D. R. An acoustic study of nasality. *Journal of Speech and Hearing Research,* 1962, **5,** 103–111.
115. DiSimoni, F. G. Evidence for a theory of speech production based on observations of the speech of children. *The Journal of the Acoustical Society of America,* 1974, **56,** 1919–1921.
116. Elliott, L. L., & Armbruster, V. B. Some possible effects of the delay of early treatment of deafness. *Journal of Speech and Hearing Research,* 1967, **10,** 209–224.
117. Elliott, L. L., & Niemoeller, A. F. The role of hearing in controlling voice fundamental frequency. *International Audiology,* 1970, **9,** 47–52.
118. Erber, N. P. Interaction of audition and vision in the recognition of aural speech stimuli. *Journal of Speech and Hearing Research,* 1969, **12,** 423–425.
119. Erber, N. P. Visual perception of speech by deaf children: Recent developments and continuing needs. *Journal of Speech and Hearing Disorders,* 1974, **39,** 178–185.
120. Fleming, K. J. Guidelines for choosing appropriate phonetic contexts for speech-sound recognition and production practice. *Journal of Speech and Hearing Disorders,* 1971, **36,** 356–367.
    Directed to speech clinicians trying to correct the articulation of clients whose hearing is presumably normal. Though the author

did not have deafness in mind, many of her ideas could be helpful to teachers of the deaf. The article summarizes the effects which neighboring sounds are likely to have on the ease or difficulty of recognizing or producing a particular "problem" sound. Lists and explains a number of general characteristics of contexts which are worthy of consideration in devising articulation and recognition exercises.

121. Foust, K. O. & Gengel, R. W. Speech discrimination by sensorineural hearing-impaired persons using a transposer hearing aid. *Scandinavian Audiology,* 1973, **2,** 161–170.

122. Fry, D. B. Acoustic cues in the speech of the hearing and the deaf. *Proceedings of the Royal Society of Medicine,* 1973, **66,** 959–969 (Section of Otology, 31–41).

123. Fujimura, O. Analysis of nasal consonants. *Journal of Speech and Hearing Disorders,* 1957, **22,** 190–204.

124. Gallaudet College. *Additional handicapping conditions among hearing impaired students: United States: 1971–1972.* Data from the Annual Survey of Hearing Impaired Children and Youth. Washington, D.C.: Gallaudet College, Office of Demographic Studies, 1973.

125. Gibson, E. J., Shurcliff, A., & Yonas, A. Utilization of spelling patterns by deaf and hearing subjects. In H. Levin & J. P. Williams (Eds.), *Basic studies on reading.* New York: Basic Books, 1970.

126. Gilbert, J. H. The learning of speechlike stimuli by children. *Journal of Experimental Child Psychology,* 1970, **9,** 1–11.

127. Goldman, R., & Dixon, S. D. The relationship of vocal-phonic and articulatory abilities. *Journal of Learning Disabilities,* 1971, **4,** 251–256.

128. Green, D. S. Fundamental frequency characteristics of the speech of profoundly deaf individuals. Doctoral dissertation, Purdue University, 1956.

129. Gruber, J. S. Playing with distinctive features in the babbling of infants. In C. A. Ferguson & D. I. Slobin (Eds.), *Studies of child language and development.* New York: Holt, Rinehart, and Winston, 1973.

130. Hirsh, I. J. Auditory perception of temporal order. *Journal of the Acoustical Society of America,* 1959, **31,** 759–767.

131. Hood, R. B. Some physical concomitants of speech rhythm of the deaf. *Proceedings of the International Conference on Oral Education of the Deaf.* Washington, D.C.: The Alexander Graham Bell Association for the Deaf, 1967, 921–925.

132. House, A. S. (Ed.). *Communicating by language: The speech process.* Proceedings of a conference, Princeton, New Jersey, 1964. Bethesda, Maryland: U.S. Department of Health, Education, and Welfare, National Institute of Child Health and Development.
Report of a conference of investigators and clinicians dealing with the perception of speech, speech behavior, the structure of the linguistic code, development and deficits in language skills, production of speech, disorders of speech production and perception, neural mechanisms and models, man-machine communication, and machine analogies of human communication.

133. Huntington, D. A., Harris, K. S., & Shankweiler, D. Some observations on monosyllable production by deaf speakers and dysarthric speakers. *American Annals of the Deaf,* 1968, **113,** 134–146.

134. Irvin, B. E., & Wilson, L. S. The voiced-unvoiced distinction in deaf speech. *American Annals of the Deaf,* 1973, **118,** 43–45.

135. Irwin, O. Infant speech: Consonantal sounds according to place of articulation. *Journal of Speech and Hearing Disorders,* 1947, **12,** 397–401.

136. Johansson, B. The use of the transposer for the management of the deaf child. *International Audiology,* 1966, **5,** 362–371.

137. John, J. E., & Howarth, J. N. The effect of time distortion on the intelligibility of deaf children's speech. *Language and Speech,* 1965, **8,** 127–134.

138. Jones, C. "Deaf voice": A description derived from a survey of the literature. *The Volta Review,* 1967, **69,** 507–508, 539–540.

139. Koenigsknecht, R. A. An investigation of the discrimination of certain spectral and temporal acoustic cues for speech sounds in three-year-old children, six-year-old children, and adults. Doctoral dissertation, Northwestern University, Evanston, Illinois, 1968.

140. Lach, R., Ling, A. H. & Ship, N. Early speech development in deaf infants. *American Annals of the Deaf,* 1970, **115,** 522–526.

141. Ladefoged, P. *Elements of acoustic phonetics.* Chicago: University of Chicago Press, 1962.
Just what the title says. No math required.

142. Lehiste, I., & Peterson, G. E. Transitions, glides, and diphthongs. *The Journal of the Acoustical Society of America,* 1961, **33,** 268–277.

143. Levitt, H. Sensory aids for the deaf: An overview. In C. P. Smith (Ed.), *Conference on Speech Communication and Processing.* Air Force Cambridge Research Laboratories, Cambridge, Massachusetts, AFCRL-72-0120. Special Report No. 131, 1972b.

144. Lieberman, P. *Intonation, perception, and language.* Cambridge, Massachusetts: Massachusetts Institute of Technology Press, 1967. (Monograph #38.)
Analysis of some linguistic aspects of intonation. Discusses in detail the breath group as both a physiological and linguistic event. Presents a theory of the development of intonation in the very young infant. Examines critically concepts which assume the existence of pitch phonemes in ladder-like levels. Chapter 9 is a critical survey of some fairly recent writings (1892–1965) about the linguistics of intonation.

145. Lisker, L., & Abramson, A. S. Some effects of context on voice onset time in English stops. *Language and Speech,* 1967, **10,** 1–28.

146. Locke, J. L. Questionable assumptions underlying articulation research. *Journal of Speech and Hearing Disorders,* 1968, **33,** 113–116.

147. Locke, J. L. The child's acquisition of phonetic behavior. *Acta Symbolica,* 1971, **2,** 28–32.

148. Locke, J. L., & Locke, V. L. Deaf children's phonetic, visual and dactylic coding in a grapheme recall task. *Journal of Experimental Psychology,* 1971, **89,** 142–146.

149. Locke, J. L., & Kutz, K. J. Memory for speech and speech for memory. *Journal of Speech and Hearing Research,* 1975, **18,** 176–191.
Suggests ways in which subvocalization may aid recall, including motor and acoustic encoding. An echoic store provides additional recall support if subjects rehearse vocally.

150. MacNeilage, P. F., & DeClerk, J. E. On the motor control of coarticulation in CVC monosyllables. *Journal of the Acoustical Society of America,* 1969, **45,** 1217–1233.
Investigated the effects of intrasyllable context on tongue movements in the speech of a normally-hearing person. Used cinefluorograms and electromyograms to observe activity of the tongue muscles. Found that motor control of a later syllable component was always influenced by the identity of an earlier component of the syllable, and that motor control of an earlier syllable component was almost always influenced by the identity of a later component. Includes considerable theoretical discussion.

151. MacNeilage, P. F., & Sholes, G. N. An electromyograph study of the tongue during vowel production. *Journal of Speech and Hearing Research,* 1964, **7,** 209–232.

152. Madison, C. L., et al. Speech-sound discrimination and tactile-kines-

thetic discrimination in reference to speech production. *Perceptive Motor Skills,* 1971, **33,** 831–838.

153. Markides, A. The speech of deaf and partially hearing children with special reference to factors affecting intelligibility. *British Journal of Disorders of Communication,* 1970, **5,** 126–140.

154. Mavilya, M. *Spontaneous vocalization and babbling in hearing impaired infants.* Doctoral dissertation, Teachers College, Columbia University, 1969.

155. McClumpha, S. *Cinefluorographic investigation of velopharyngeal function in selected deaf speakers.* Master of Arts thesis, University of Florida, 1966.

156. McReynolds, L.V., & Houston, K. A distinctive feature analysis of children's misarticulations. *Journal of Speech and Hearing Disorders,* 1971, **36,** 155–166.

157. Menyuk, P. The role of distinctive features in children's acquisition of phonology. *Journal of Speech and Hearing Research,* 1968, **11,** 138–146.

158. Menyuk, P. *The development of speech.* Indianapolis: Bobbs-Merrill, 1972. (44 pages, 55 references.)

159. Miller, J. D. Directions for research to improve hearing aids and services for the hearing-impaired. *A report of Working Group 65, NAS-NRC, Committee on Hearing, Bioacoustics, and Biomechanics.* Washington, D.C.: National Academy of Science, 1972.

160. Moll, K. L. Velopharyngeal closure on vowels. *Journal of Speech and Hearing Research,* 1962, **5,** 30–37.
Using cinefluorographs of normally-hearing speakers, the variations in velopharyngeal closure in vowels as a function of the context of the vowels were measured. Concluded that the low vowels exhibit less closure than the high vowels; that vowels adjacent to /n/ exhibit incomplete closure, with the vowels preceding /n/ having less closure than those following /n/; and that there are no significant differences between the effects of various non-nasal contexts on vowel closure, but there is a tendency for less closure on isolated vowels than on vowels in non-nasal consonant contexts.

161. Moll, K. L., & Daniloff, R. G. Investigation of the timing of velar movements during speech. *Journal of the Acoustical Society of America,* 1971, **50,** 671–684.
Investigates coarticulation in the speech of normally-hearing persons by cinefluorographic observations of movements of the velum

during spoken sentences. Found that where velum movement is required for the articulation of a phoneme, the velum may start to move toward the required position several syllables in anticipation of the actual production of the phoneme. The authors discuss a theory of coarticulation which they think may explain their findings.

162. Monaghan, A. The need for a school to have a philosophy of teaching speech. *The Volta Review*, 1958, **60,** 386–391.

163. Monsen, R. Personal Communication.

164. Morkovin, B. V. Organic and inhibitory factors of speech production disturbances in children with hearing disorders. *Report of Proceedings of the International Congress on Education of the Deaf and the 41st Meeting of the Convention of American Instructors of the Deaf, 1963*. Washington, D.C.: U.S. Government Printing Office, 1964, 726–734.

165. Morkovin, B. V. Language in the general development of the preschool deaf child: A review of research in the Soviet Union. *ASHA: Journal of the American Speech and Hearing Association*, 1968, **10,** 195–199.
    Discusses research of the Moscow Institute of Defectology directed toward developing the speech, language, intellects, and personalities of deaf children. References are listed, although the research itself is not described. Among the facets of the MID's approach which the author discusses are: fingerspelling, used to launch little deaf children into language, but eventually to be replaced by lipreading and speech; an enriched environment of child-center experiences in which both verbal and nonverbal communication are encouraged; and formal classes in which lipreading, articulation, grammar, etc., are taught.

166. Moskowitz, A. I. The two-year-old stage in the acquisition of English phonology. *Language*, 1970, **46,** 426–441.

167. Mowrer, D. Transfer of training in articulation therapy. *Journal of Speech and Hearing Disorders*, 1971, **36,** 427–466.

168. Nickerson, R. S. Characteristics of the speech of deaf persons. *The Volta Review*, 1975, **77,** 342–362.

169. Niemoeller, A. F. Acoustical design of classrooms for the deaf. *American Annals of the Deaf*, 1968, **113,** 1040–1045.

170. Northcott, W. H. (Ed.) *The hearing impaired child in a regular classroom: Preschool, elementary, and secondary years*. Washington, D.C.: The Alexander Graham Bell Association for the Deaf, 1973.

171. *Oral sensation and perception: Proceedings of a symposium.* Springfield, Illinois: Charles C Thomas, 1969.
172. Oyer, H. J. *Auditory communication for the hard of hearing.* Englewood Cliffs, N.J.: Prentice-Hall, Inc., 1966.
173. Parker, A. The laryngograph. *Hearing* (The Royal National Institute for the Deaf), 1974, **29,** 256–261.
174. Phillips, J. R. Formal characteristics of speech which mothers address to their young children. Doctoral dissertation, The Johns Hopkins University, Baltimore, Maryland, 1970.
175. Pickett, J. M. Some applications of speech analysis to communication aids for the deaf. *The Volta Review,* 1971, **73,** 147–156.
      A description of several tactual and visual speech aids.

176. Pickett, J. M., & Pickett, R. H. Communication of speech sounds by a tactual vocoder. *Journal of Speech and Hearing Research,* 1963, **6,** 207–222.
      Discusses results of speech perception tests when the speech signal was analyzed into 10 frequency bands of energy, each of which was presented as vibrations to a different finger of the "listener's" hands. All 10 vibrators had a frequency of 300 Hz, but each differed from the other in vibration amplitude according to the energy distribution among the various frequency bands of the original speech.

177. Pitman, J. Can I.T.A. help the deaf child, his parents, and his teacher? In *Proceedings of the International Conference on Oral Education of the Deaf.* Washington, D.C.: The Alexander Graham Bell Association for the Deaf, 1967, 514–542.
      The father of the Initial Teaching Alphabet argues that it should be used in the teaching of deaf children, including infants. He suggests that World I.T.A., rather than standard I.T.A., would be more suitable, because the World version provides some information about stress and about vowel neutralization.

178. Potter, R. K., Kopp, G. A., & Green, H. C. *Visible speech.* New York: Van Nostrand, 1947.
179. Preston, M. S., Yeni-Komshian, G., Stark, R. E., & Port, D. K. Certain aspects of speech production and perception in children (Abstract). *Journal of the Acoustical Society of America,* 1969, **46,** 102.
180. Prosek, R. A., & House, A. S. Intraoral air pressure as a feedback cue in consonant production. *Journal of Speech and Hearing Research,* 1975, **18,** 133–147.

181. Rebelsky, F., & Hanks, C. Fathers' verbal interaction with infants in the first three months of life. *Child Development*, 1971, **42**, 63–68.

182. Risberg, A. A critical review of work on speech analyzing hearing aids. *The Volta Review*, 1971, **73**, 23–32.

183. Sander, E. K. When are speech sounds learned? *Journal of Speech and Hearing Disorders*, 1972, **37**, 55–63.

184. Schour, I., & Massler, M. The development of the human dentition. *The Journal of the American Dental Association*, 1941, **28**, 1153–1160.

185. Schunhoff, H. F. (Ed.) *The teaching of speech and by speech in public residential schools for the deaf in the United States, 1815–1955.* Romney, W. Va.: West Virginia Schools for the Deaf and the Blind, 1957.

186. Sheppard, W. C., & Lane, H. L. Development of the prosodic features of infant vocalizing. *Journal of Speech and Hearing Research*, 1968, **11**, 94–108.

187. Silverman, S. R. Tolerance for pure tones and speech in normal and defective hearing. *Annals of Otology*, 1947, **56**, 658–678.
    A summary of studies that dealt with the mapping of thresholds of discomfort and pain in listening to loud sounds.

188. Slis, I. H., & Cohen, A. On the complex regulating the voiced-voiceless distinction II. *Language and Speech*, 1969, **12**, 137–155.

189. Smith, C. Residual hearing and speech production in deaf children. *Communicative Sciences Laboratory Report #4*. New York: City University of New York Graduate Center, 1973.

190. Snow, C. E. Mother's speech to children learning language. *Child Development*, 1973, **43**, 549–565.

191. Stark, R. E. (Ed.) *Sensory capabilities of hearing-impaired children.* Baltimore, Maryland: University Park Press, 1974.
    Proceedings of a workshop of speech and hearing scientists and workers on speech of hearing impaired children dealing with the needs and capabilities of children for whom auditory and non-auditory aids were being designed. The topics included sensory capabilities, perceptual and cognitive strategies, and language processing.

192. Stark, R., Tallal, P., & Curtiss, B. Speech perception and production errors in dysphasic children. *Journal of the Acoustical Society of America*, 1975, **57**, Supplement 1, 524.
    An abstract of studies demonstrating that dysphasics who failed to discriminate between speech sounds which incorporate brief duration acoustic cues also failed to produce such speech sounds correctly.

193. Stetson, R. H. *Motor phonetics.* Amsterdam, Holland: North Holland Publishing Co., 1951.

194. Stevens, K. N., & House, A. S. Perturbation of vowel articulations by consonantal context: An acoustical study. *Journal of Speech and Hearing Research,* 1963, **6,** 111–128.

195. Stevens, K. N., & Klatt, D. H. Role of formant transitions in the voiced-voiceless distinction for stops. *Journal of the Acoustical Society of America,* 1974, **55,** 653–659.

196. Stewart, R. B. By ear alone. *American Annals of the Deaf,* 1968, **113,** 147–155.

197. Suchman, R. G. Visual impairment among deaf children. *Archives of Ophthalmology,* 1967, **77,** 18–21.

198. Swets, A., & Elliott, L. (Eds.). *Psychology and the handicapped child.* Washington, D.C.: U.S. Department of Health, Education and Welfare, 1974.

199. Thomas, W. G. Intelligibility of the speech of deaf children. *Report of Proceedings of the International Congress on Education of the Deaf and the 41st Meeting of the Convention of American Instructors of the Deaf, 1963.* Washington, D.C.: U.S. Government Printing Office, 1964. (Document 106, 245–261.)
    Evaluates the effects on the intelligibility of the speech of deaf children of three factors: the kind of speech materials; whether or not the listener could see the speaker; and the previous experience of the listener with deaf children.

200. Travis, L. E. (Ed.) *Handbook of speech pathology and audiology.* New York: Appleton-Century-Crofts, 1971.
    A massive reference work of more than 1300 pages containing much fundamental information on speech production. The bibliographies are impressively extensive.

201. Tervoort, B. Speech and language development in the normal and hearing impaired child (Dutch). *Gehoorgestoorde Kind,* 1973, **13,** 77–87.

202. Vegeley, C. Monitoring of monosyllabic words by deaf children. *Report of Proceedings of the International Congress on Education of the Deaf and the 41st Meeting of the Convention of American Instructors of the Deaf, 1963.* Washington, D.C.: U.S. Government Printing Office, 1964. (Document 106, 735–748.)
    Evaluation of the intelligibility of deaf talkers' speech by the deaf speakers themselves and also by normally-hearing listeners.

203. Voelker, C. H. An experimental study of the comparative rate of utterance of deaf and normal hearing speakers. *American Annals of the Deaf,* 1938, **83,** 274–284.

204. Webster, R. L. Changes in infants' vocalizations as a function of differential acoustic stimulation. *Developmental Psychology,* 1972, **7,** 39–43.

205. Weiner, P. S. Auditory discrimination and articulation. *Journal of Speech and Hearing Disorders,* 1967, **32,** 19–28.

   A survey of published research which bears on the question of whether or not presumably normally-hearing persons who make articulation errors in their own speech also tend to make errors in distinguishing among the speech sounds spoken by others. Discusses a number of the variables which affect this relation.

206. Willemain, T. R., & Lee, F. F. Tactile pitch feedback for deaf speakers. *The Volta Review,* 1971, **73,** 541–553.

   Describes a device which pokes different fingers of a speaker's hand to signal him that his pitch is too high, too low, or satisfactory. A hypothesis to explain the cause of unnaturally high pitch in the speech of the deaf is offered.

207. Wilson, D. K. *Voice problems of children.* Baltimore, Maryland: The Williams and Wilkins Co., 1972.

208. Winitz, H. *Articulatory acquisition and behavior.* New York: Appleton-Century-Crofts, 1969

   A book attempting to "bring articulation, as studied by the speech pathologist, within the mainstream of present-day psycholinguistic thought." Methods and models of descriptive linguistics, instrumental phonetics, and learning theory related to articulatory behavior and correction.

209. Wolfe, W. D., & Goulding, D. J. (Eds.) *Articulation and learning.* Springfield, Illinois: Charles C Thomas, 1973.

SECTION C.
MORE RESEARCH AND GENERAL BACKGROUND

210. Brodnitz, F. S. Semantics of the voice. *Journal of Speech and Hearing Disorders,* 1967, **32,** 325–330.

211. Brown, R. *A first language: The early stages.* Cambridge, Massachusetts: Harvard University Press, 1973.

   Draws on psychology and linguistics to treat first stages of language acquisition. Starts with the threshold of syntax when children begin to combine words to make sentences and then moves on to modulations of basic structural meanings and acquisition of morphemes.

212. Brown, R., & Bellugi, U. Three processes in the child's acquisition of syntax. *Harvard Education Review,* 1964, **34,** 133–151.

213. Cazden, C. B. Some implications of research on language development for preschool education. In R. D. Hess & R. M. Bear (Eds.), *Early education: Current theory, research and practice.* Chicago: Aldine Press, 1967.

214. Cooper, F. S., Abramson, A. S., Swashima, M., & Lisker, L. Looking at the larynx during running speech. *Annals of Otology, Rhinology, and Laryngology,* 1971, **80,** 678–682.

215. Cruttenden, A. A phonetic study of babbling. *British Journal of Communication Disorders,* 1970, **5,** 110–117.

216. Denes, P. B., & Pinson, E. N. *The speech chain.* New York: Bell Telephone Laboratories, Inc., 1963. New York: Doubleday, 1973.
    An easy to understand, simplified but accurate account of communication by speech and hearing, including linguistics, physiology, anatomy, and acoustics.

217. Eguchi, S., & Hirsh, I. J. Development of speech sounds in children. *Acta Oto-Laryngologica,* 1969, Supplement, **257,** 5–51.
    Spectrographic analysis of changes in the accuracy of phonemes in the speech of normally-hearing children as their ages increased from 3 to 13 years old. These normally-hearing children's precision of timing in a plosive-vowel syllable did not reach a maximum until about age 9; accuracy of the children's vowels reached a maximum by about age 11.

218. Eimas, P. D., Siqueland, E. R., Jusczyk, P., et al. Speech perception in infants. *Science,* 1971, **171,** 303–306.

219. Farb, P. *Word play: What happens when people talk.* New York: Alfred A. Knopf, 1974.
    A popular treatise on speech and language and their relation to human behavior. Draws on work of modern linguists.

220. Francis, H. Structure in the speech of a two-and-a-half-year-old. *British Journal of Educational Psychology,* 1969, **39,** 291–302.

221. Fry, D. B. Phonemic system in children's speech. *British Journal of Communication Disorders,* 1968, **3,** 13–19.

222. Gay, T., & Harris, K. S. Some recent developments in the use of elec-

tromyography in speech research. *Journal of Speech and Hearing Research,* 1971, **14,** 241–246.

223. Geldard, F. A. Pattern perception by the skin. In D. R. Kenshalo (Ed.), *The skin senses.* Springfield, Illinois: Charles C Thomas, 1968.

224. Gilbert, J. H. Formant concentration positions in the speech of children at two levels of linguistic development. *Journal of the Acoustical Society of America,* 1970, **48** (Part 2), 1404–1406.

Shows no significant difference in vowel production accuracy between 4-year-olds with normal language development and 4-year-olds with retarded language development. Both groups of children had normal hearing.

225. Graham, L. W., & House, A. S. Phonological oppositions in children: A perceptual study. *Journal of the Acoustical Society of America,* 1971, **49** (Part 2), 559–566.

Investigation of the ability of normally-hearing 3- to 4-1/2-year-olds to tell whether the members of various pairs of speech sounds were both the same or were different. Discusses the relevance of several linguistic classification systems to the problem of understanding the actual process of perceiving differences between sounds.

226. Gray, W. G., & Wise, C. M. *The bases of speech* (3rd Ed.) New York: Harper and Brothers, 1959.

A textbook on speech. Not specifically concerned with the speech of the deaf, but encompasses it. Provides basic information on the nature of speech from the points of view of its social basis, its genesis, physics, physiology and neurology, psychology, phonetics, linguistics, and semantics.

227. Greenberg, S. R. *An experimental study of certain intonation contrasts in American English.* Working Papers in Phonetics No. 13. Los Angeles, California: University of California (Los Angeles) Press, 1969.

228. Haber, R. N., & Hershenson, M. *The psychology of visual perception.* New York: Holt, Rinehart, and Winston, 1973.

229. Hilgard, E. R. *Theories of learning* (2nd ed.) New York: Appleton-Century-Crofts, Inc., 1956. (Pp. 486–487.)

230. Hirsh, I. J., & Sherrick, C. E. Perceived order in different sense modalities. *Journal of Experimental Psychology,* 1961, **62,** 423–432.

231. Ingraw, D. Phonological rules in young children. *Papers and Reports on Child Language Development, Committee on Linguistics, Stanford University, 1971,* **3,** 31–50.

232. Jakobson, R. C., & Halle, M. *Fundamentals of language.* 'S-Grav-enhage, The Netherlands: Mouton and Co., 1956.
Early statement of "distinctive features" of speech by two promi-nent scholars in linguistics.

233. Jakobson, R. C., Fant, G. M., & Halle, M. *Preliminaries to speech anal-ysis: The distinctive features and their correlates.* Cambridge, Massachusetts: Massachusetts Institute of Technology Press, 1969.
Fundamental up-to-date treatment of "distinctive features."

234. Jones, S. J., & Moss, H. A. Age, state, and maternal behavior asso-ciated with infant vocalizations. *Child Development,* 1971, **42,** 1039–1051.

235. Kantner, C. E., West, R., & Wise, H. S. *Phonetics* (Rev. ed.) New York: Harper and Brothers, 1960.
A basic reference and textbook for an introductory phonetics course. Includes phonetic transcription and analysis of phonemes, with particular attention to shades of differences in pronunciation resulting from coarticulation.

236. Kaplan, E. L. The role of intonation in the acquisition of language. Doc-toral dissertation, Cornell University, Ithaca, New York, 1969.

237. Kaplan, E., & Kaplan, G. The prelinguistic child. In J. Eliot (Ed.), *Hu-man development and cognitive processes.* New York: Holt, Rine-hart, and Winston, 1971.

238. Kellog, W. N. Communication and language in the home-raised chim-panzee. *Science,* 1968, **162,** 423–427.

239. Laubach, F. C., Kirk, E. M., & Laubach, R. S. *The new stream-lined English series: Teachers' manual.* Syracuse, New York: New Readers Press, 1971.

240. Lehiste, I., & Peterson, G. E. Transitions, glides, and diphthongs. *Jour-nal of the Acoustical Society of America,* 1961, **33,** 268–277.

241. Lenneberg, E. H., & Long, B. S. Language development. *Psychology and the Handicapped Child* (U.S. Department of Health, Educa-tion, and Welfare). Washington, D.C.: U.S. Government Printing Office, 1974, No. (OE) 73-05000, 127-148.)

242. Liakh, G. S. Imitation of articulatory movements and of sound produc-tion in early infancy. *Neuroscience Transactions,* 1969, **8,** 913–917.

243. Liberman, A. M. The grammars of speech and language. *Cognitive Psy-chology,* 1970, **1,** 301–323.

244. Liberman, A. M., et al. A motor theory of speech perception. *Proceed-

ings of Speech Communication Seminar, 1962. Stockholm, Sweden: Royal Institute of Technology, Transmission Laboratory, 1963.

Argues for a theory that the perceived distinctiveness of a phoneme is tightly linked to the listener's associating the acoustic signal with the articulatory movements appropriate for the phoneme.

245. Malmberg, R. (Ed.) *Manual of phonetics.* Amsterdam, Holland: North Holland Publishing Co., 1920.

A scientific and current treatment of phonetics. The subjects include the linguistic basis of phonetics; acoustical foundations of phonetics; the functional anatomy of the speech organs; the auditory basis of phonetics; the psychological basis of phonetics; statistical methods in phonetics; the speech communication process; analysis and synthesis of speech processes; mechanism of the larynx and the laryngeal vibrations; the articulatory possibilities of man; radiographic, palatographic, and labiographic methods in phonetics; prosodic phenomena; phonology in relation to phonetics; phonotactic aspects of the linguistic expression; phonetics and linguistic evolution; phonetics and sociology; phonetics and pathology; and phonetics in its relation to aesthetics.

246. Martin, J. G. Rhythmic (hierarchical) versus serial structure in speech and other behavior. *Psychological Review,* 1972, **79,** 487–509.

247. McElroy, C. W. *Speech and language development of the preschool child.* Springfield, Illinois: Charles C Thomas, 1972.

248. Miller, G. A., & Nicely, P. E. Analysis of perceptual confusions among some English consonants. *Journal of the Acoustical Society of America,* 1955, **27,** 338–352.

Summary of research which analyzed the kinds of consonant confusions that normally-hearing listeners tend to make in listening to speech in noise and distorted by deletion of various frequencies. The task of the listeners in this experiment was somewhat analogous to the task faced by hearing impaired persons receiving normal speech. The experimenters grouped their test consonants according to similarity in the features of voicing, nasality, affrication, duration, and place of articulation. Confusion matrices provide a basis for inferring which of these features are likely to become equivocal under various conditions of signal to noise ratio and frequency loss.

249. Morse, P. A. The discrimination of speech and nonspeech stimuli in early infancy. *Journal of Experimental Child Psychology,* 1972, **14,** 477–492.

250. Nakazima, S. A comparative study of the speech developments of Japanese and American English in childhood: The reorganization process of babbling articulation mechanisms. *Studies in Phonology,* 1970, **5,** 20–36.

251. Nash, J. *Developmental psychology: A psychobiological approach.* Englewood Cliffs, New Jersey: Prentice-Hall, Inc., 1970.
    Proceeds from a description of the biology of human development to a discussion of the environment's interaction with this biological basis. Of particular interest is the treatment of critical periods in development, early stimulation, development of the capacity for learning, and development of communication and cognitive processes.

252. Perkins, W. H. *Speech pathology: An applied behavioral science.* St. Louis, Missouri: Mosby Press, 1971.
    A "behavioral science" approach to speech pathology for the beginning student, logically organized and built around questions frequently raised by students and others. A good synthesis of ideas on the development of speech. Good bibliography.

253. Peterson, G. E., & Barney, H. L. Control methods used in a study of vowels. *Journal of the Acoustical Society of America,* 1952, **24,** 175–184.

254. Peterson, G. E., & Shoup, J. E. A physiological theory of phonetics. *Journal of Speech and Hearing Research,* 1966, **9,** 5–67.
    Draws together the definitions, assumptions, and concepts about speech and the physiological mechanism for producing it which, in the authors' opinion, are required for accurately, completely, and unequivocally describing any speech sound in any language in terms of the physiological events and conditions necessary for the production of that sound. A set of universally applicable symbols for phonetic notation is defined by being arrayed in charts which list the physiological parameters of speech as identified by the authors. Includes much philosophy about theoretical models of highly complex systems such as a phonetic system.

255. Peterson, G. E., & Shoup, J. E. The elements of an acoustic phonetic theory. *Journal of Speech and Hearing Research,* 1966, **9,** 68–99.
    A definition of the acoustic characteristics of speech and a sum-

mary of the relationships of these characteristics to physiological phonetics and descriptive phonetics.

256. Peterson, G. E., & Shoup, J. E. Glossary of terms from the physiological and acoustical phonetic theories. *Journal of Speech and Hearing Research,* 1966, **9,** 100–120.
An alphabetically arranged summary of definitions from related references by same authors.

257. Pike, K. L. *The intonation of American English.* Ann Arbor, Michigan: The University of Michigan Press, 1945.

258. Pollack, I. Within-and-between-modality correlation detection. *Journal of the Acoustical Society of America,* 1974, **55,** 641–644.

259. Stevenson, H. W. *Children's learning.* Englewood Cliffs, New Jersey: Prentice Hall, Inc., 1972.
A recent research-based treatment of children's learning. Of particular interest are Chapters 4 through 10 concerned with language and learning and Chapter 19 on perceptual learning. The role of reinforcement is analyzed as it influences learning in various task contexts.

260. Todd, G., & Palmer, B. Social reinforcement of infant babbling. *Child Development,* 1968, **39,** 591–596.

261. Trehub, S. E., & Rabinovitch, M. S. Auditory-linguistic sensitivity in early infancy. *Developmental Psychology,* 1972, **6,** 74–77.

262. Venezky, R. L. English orthography: Its graphical structure and its relation to sound. *Reading Research Quarterly,* 1967, **2,** 75–105.
Concepts about spelling which lead to regular relationships between the pronunciation and spelling of English words, many of which would ordinarily be considered hopelessly irregular. The author's insight into the regular patterns apparently embedded in the complex of spelling-meaning-pronunciation was aided by a computer assisted analysis of 20,000 common English words. Inspires respect for the learning and skill of the ordinary reader who can, with reasonable correctness, pronounce new words that he encounters in his reading.

263. Waterson, N. Child phonology: A prosodic view. *Journal of Linguistics,* 1971, **7,** 179–211.

264. Zipf, G. K. *The psycho-biology of language: An introduction to dynamic philology.* Cambridge, Massachusetts: The Massachusetts Institute of Technology Press, 1965.
A book of fascinating insights and theories about speech and lan-

guage approached through statistical analysis. For example, Chapter III, "The Form and Behavior of Phonemes," after a clear and interesting discussion of the concept of phoneme, builds and ties together a complex of theories about the frequency of occurrence of phonemes and words, the complexity and effort of production, and phonological evolution. First published in 1935, the present edition is enhanced by an introduction by G. A. Miller in which he puts much of Zipf's theorizing into perspective.

265. Zubek, J. P. (Ed.) *Sensory deprivation: Fifteen years of research.* New York: Appleton-Century-Crofts, 1969.

A review of research of sensory deprivation. Most of the research reviewed involved contrived laboratory situations using normal adult subjects. Does not enter the realm of deafness and only fleetingly alludes to the effects of sensory deprivation on children. Nevertheless, a central idea to which the bulk of the book points—that sensory stimulation is important for the maintenance of effective functioning—is of interest to those concerned with the education of the deaf.

Index of Names

A

Abramson, A.S.	223, 230
Adams, R.E.	203
Alcorn, S.K.	202
Anderson, D.C.	214
Angelocci, A.A.	202
Archambault, P.	203
Armbruster, V.B.	220
Avery, C.B.	203
Avondino, J.	203

B

Barney, H.L.	234
Bass, S.	214
Bear, R.M.	154, 230
Becking, A.G.T.	218
Beckwith, L.	218
Beebe, H.H.	83, 148, 203
Bell, A.M.	9, 215
Bell, A.G.	9, 15, 203, 217
Bellugi, U.	154, 230
Berg, F.S.	206
Bishop, M.E.	46, 218
Black, J.W.	218
Blanton, R.L.	218
Blasdell, R.	219
Boothroyd, A.	203, 219
Børrild, K.	213
Brannon, J.B., Jr.	219
Brodnitz, F.S.	229
Brown, R.	154, 229, 230

C

California State Master Plan for Education of the Deaf	167, 219
Calvert, D.R.	55, 182, 186, 190, 203, 206, 219
Carr, J.	206, 219
Cazden, C.B.	154, 230

Chase, R.	213
Chen, M.	219
Clarke School for the Deaf	83, 117, 204
Cohen, A.	227
Cohen, M.L.	214, 219
Colton, R.H.	219
Connor, L.E.	204
Conrad, R.	220
Constam, A.	214
Cooker, H.S.	219
Cooper, F.S.	213, 230
Cornett, R.O.	204
Crawford, G.H.	208
Cruttenden, A.	230
Cullen, J.K. Jr.	213
Curtiss, B.	227

D

Daniloff, R.G.	224
Davis, H.	151, 220
DeClerk, J.E.	223
Denes, P.B.	220, 230
DiCarlo, L.S.	204
Dickson, D.R.	220
DiSimoni, F.G.	220
Dixon, S.D.	221
Doehring, D.G.	72, 204

E

Eguchi, S.	230
Eilers, R.E.	204
Eimas, P.D.	230
Eliot, J.	232
Elliott, L.L.	220, 228
Erber, N.P.	204, 220
Ewing, A.	205, 217
Ewing, E.C.	205
Ewing, I.R.	205

F

Fairbanks, G.	37, 205
Fant, G.M.	211, 232
Farb, P.	230
Fellendorf, G.	205
Ferguson, C.A.	221
Fleming, K.J.	220
Fletcher, S.G.	206
Foust, K.O.	221
Francis, H.	230
French, S.L.	206
Fry, D.B.	206, 217, 221, 230
Fujimura, O.	221
Funderburg, R.S.	211

G

Gallaudet College Office of Demographic Studies	5, 44, 148, 167, 211, 221
Gault, R.H.	206
Gay, T.	230
Geers, A.V.	viii, 170, 197
Geldard, F.A.	231
Gengel, R.W.	221
Gibson, E.J.	221
Gilbert, J.H.	221, 231
Gjerdingen, D.	197
Goldman, R.	221
Goldstein, M.A.	83, 207
Goulding, D.J.	229
Graham, L.W.	231
Gray, W.G.	231
Green, D.S.	186, 221
Green, H.C.	226
Greenberg, S.R.	231
Greer, C.W.	204
Griffiths, C.	148, 207
Gruber, J.S.	221
Gruver, M.H.	202, 207
Guberina, P.	207
Guttman, N.	214

H

Haber, R.N.	231
Halle, M.	232
Hanks, C.	227
Harrell, H.	206
Harris, K.S.	222, 230
Haycock, G.S.	207
Hershenson, M.	231
Hess, R.D.	154, 230
Hilgard, E.R.	48, 231
Hirsh, I.J.	208, 221, 230, 231
Holbrook, A.	208

Hood, R.B.	187, 221
House, A.S.	46, 150, 218, 222, 226, 228, 231
Houston, K.	224
Howarth, J.N.	222
Hudgins, C.V.	161, 177, 187, 209, 210
Huntington, D.A.	222

I

Ingraw, D.	231
Irvin, B.E.	222
Irwin, O.	222

J

Jakobson, R.C.	232
Jeffers, J.	210
Jensen, P.	219
Johansson, B.	222
John, J.E.	222
John Tracy Clinic	210
Joiner, E.	210
Jones, C.	222
Jones, S.J.	232
Jusczyk, P.	230

K

Kantner, C.E.	232
Kaplan, E.L.	232
Kaplan, G.	232
Kellogg, W.N.	232
Kelly, J.C.	83, 211
Kenshalo, D.R.	231
Kirk, E.M.	14, 232
Klatt, D.H.	228
Koenigsknecht, R.A.	222
Kopp, G.A.	226
Krijnen, A.	206
Kringelbotn, M.	214
Kutz, K.J.	223

L

Lach, R.	222
Ladefoged, P.	23, 222
Lane, H.L.	227
Laubach, F.C.	14, 232
Laubach, R.S.	14, 232
Laurentine, M.	211
Lee, F.F.	229
Lehiste, I.	222, 232
Lenneberg, E.H.	43, 232
Leshin, G.	211
Levin, H.	221
Levitt, H.	63, 211, 222
Liakh, G.S.	232

Liberman, A.M. 213, 232
Lieberman, P. 223
Ling, A.H. 222
Ling, D. viii, 5, 45, 64-88, 72, 89, 148, 149, 151, 157, 161, 204, 211, 214
Lisker, L. 223, 230
Locke, J.L. 223
Locke, V.L. 223
Long, B.S. 43, 232
Lorenz, M.L. 206
Lyon, E. 211

M

MacNeilage, P.F. 223
Madison, C.L. 223
Magner, M.E. 211
Malmberg, R. 23, 233
Markides, A. 224
Martin, J.G. 233
Mártony, J. 211, 213
Massler, M. 17, 227
Mavilya, M. 224
McClumpha, S. 184, 224
McElroy, C.W. 233
McGinnis, M.A. 163, 211
McReynolds, L.V. 224
Menyuk, P. 224
Miller, G.A. 206, 208, 233, 236
Miller, J.D. viii, 38, 224
Minifie, F.D. 204
Moll, K.L. 224
Monaghan, A. 225
Monsen, R. viii, 193, 225
Moog, J.S. viii, 170, 197, 211
Moores, D.F. 212
Morkovin, B.V. 225
Morse, P.A. 234
Moskowitz, A.I. 225
Moss, H.A. 232
Mowrer, D. 225
Mumford, L. vii

N

Nakazima, S. 234
Nash, J. 234
Nelson, R. 214
New, M.C. 212
Nicely, P.E. 233
Nicholas, M. 206
Nickerson, R.S. 225
Niemoeller, A.F. 220, 225
Northcott, W.H. 225
Numbers, F.C. 161, 177, 187, 209

Numbers, M.E. 205, 212
Nunnally, J.C. 218
Nye, P.W. 63, 211

O

Odom, P.B. 218
Oyer, H.J. 226

P

Palmer, B. 235
Parker, A. 226
Pearce, M.F. 211
Pennsylvania School for the Deaf 117
Perkins, W.H. 234
Peterson, G.E. 222, 232, 234, 235
Phillips, J.R. 226
Phillips, N.D. 214
Pickett, J.M. 212, 213, 214, 226
Pickett, R.H. 63, 226
Pike, K.L. 235
Pinson, E.N. 230
Pitman, J. 226
Pollack, D. 83, 148, 214
Pollack, I. 235
Port, D.K. 226
Porter, J. 215
Potter, R.K. 226
Poulos, T.H. 214
Preston, M.S. 226
Pronovost, W. 214
Prosek, R.A. 226
Pugh, B. 214

R

Rabinovitch, M.S. 235
Rebelsky, F. 227
Remillard, W. 214
Ringel, R.L. 46, 218
Risberg, A. 213, 227
Rockey, D. 163, 214
Ronnei, E.C. 215
Round Hill Round Table 215
Rozanska, E.v.D. 206

S

Sander, E.K. 227
Schmaehl, O. 206
Schour, I. 17, 227
Schunhoff, H.F. 227
Shankweiler, D.P. 213, 222
Sheppard, W.C. 227
Sherrick, C.E. 231
Ship, N. 222

Sholes, G.N. 223
Shoup, J.E. 234, 235
Shurcliff, A. 221
Silverman, S.R. 151, 215, 220, 227
Simmons, A.A. 215
Simmons,-Martin, A.A. viii, 148, 154, 155, 215
Siqueland, E.R. 230
Slis, I.H. 227
Slobin, D.I. 221
Smith, C.P. 219, 222, 227
Smith, F. 206, 208
Snow, C.E. 227
Stark, R.E. 63, 213, 215, 226, 227
Stetson, R.H. 215, 228
Stevens, K.N. 150, 228
Stevenson, H.W. 235
Stewart, R.B. 213, 228
Stoner, M. 216
Storm, R.D. 203
Studdert-Kennedy, M. 213
Suchman, R.G. 45, 228
Swashima, M. 230
Sweet, M.E. 216
Swets, A. 228

T

Tallal, P. 227
Tervoort, B. 228
Thomas, W.G. 228
Thomasia, M. 206
Todd, G. 235
Travis, L.E. 184, 228
Trehub, S.E. 235

U

Utley, J. 83, 216

V

van Uden, A. 216

Vegeley, C. 46, 50, 158, 228
Venezky, R.L. 235
Vivian, R.M. 216
Voelker, C.H. 229
Vorce, E. 217

W

Walter, B. 217
Waterson, N. 235
Watson, T.J. 217
Webster, R.L. 229
Wedenberg, E. 217
Weiner, P.S. 229
West, R. 232
Whetnall, E. 217
Whitehurst, M.W. 83, 217
Willemain, T.R. 229
Williams, J.P. 221
Wilson, D.K. 229
Wilson, L.S. 222
Winitz, H. 229
Wise, C.M. 231
Wise, H.S. 232
Wolfe, W.D. 229
Woodward, H.M.E. 206
Worcester, A. 11

Y

Yale, C.A. 11, 22, 217, 218
Yeni-Komshian, G. 226
Yenkin, L. 214
Yonas, A. 221

Z

Zaliouk, A. 9, 15, 218
Zeiser, M.L. 204
Zipf, G.K. 235
Zubek, J.P. 236

Index of Subjects

-a- 139
Abutting Consonants 182-183
Accent 34-35
a-e 145
Affricates 21
Allophone 7
Amplification (see Hearing Aids)
Antiformants 75
a(r) 142
Articulation 7-28
  Development of 160-162
  Errors of 177-183
  Manner of Production 20-23
    Affricates 21
    Fricatives 20-21
    Resonants 22
    Stops 20
  Perceptual Features of 23-27
  Place of Production 15-20
    Alveolar Ridge 18
    Lips 15
    Nasal Cavity 19
    Oral Cavity 18
    Palate 18
    Pharynx 19
    Teeth 16-17
    Tongue 18-19
Assessment 168-172
  Reviewing Results 192-195
Association Phoneme Unit Method 163-166
Auditory Feature Information and Recognition 23-26, 31, 73-77
  Frication 76
  Manner 38
  Nasality 75-76
  Onset Characteristics 76
  Pitch 38
  Place 38, 76-77
  Voicing 74-75
aw 141

b 114
Blends 182-183
Breathiness 185

Carry-over 51-52, 173
ch 110
Clusters, Consonants 182-183
Coarticulation 27-28
Consonants and Vowels, Instructional Analysis of 89-146

-a- 139	$\overset{1}{oo}$ 141
a-e 145	$\overset{2}{oo}$ 141
a(r) 142	ou 145
aw 141	p 94
b 114	qu 138
ch 110	r 135
d 116	$\overset{1}{s}$ 105
-e- 139	sh 108
ee 139	t 96
f 102	$\overset{1}{th}$ 104
g 118	$\overset{2}{th}$ 122
h 91	-u- 142
-i- 139	u-e 145
i-e 145	ur 143
j 127	v 121
k 99	w 112
l 133	wh 93
m 128	x 138
n 130	y- 137
ng 131	z 124
o-e 145	zh 125
oi 145	

d 116
Dental Occlusion 42
Deviations of Speech 175-190
  Abnormalities of Voice 183-186, 190

Correcting   175-177
Errors of Articulation   177-183
Irregularities of Rhythm   186-190
Signaling   175
Specifying   175
Diacritical Markings   10-11
Dialects   7
Difference Limen   32
Dynamic Range, Hearing   65

-e-   139
Ear Molds   82
ee   139
Emphasis   34
Environment   50-52
  Carry-over   51-52
  Language Generating Experiences   50-51
  Oral Environment   51, 52-53
Evaluation   56

f   102
Feedback   23-26
Formants   22, 69-72, 74-78
Frequency Range, Hearing Aids   68-73
Frication   76
Fricatives   20-21
Fundamental Frequency, Voice   29, 68, 186

g   118
Gain, Hearing Aids   65-67, 79-81

h   91
Harmonics, Voice   30
Hearing Aids   64-73, 78-81
  Acoustics Cues and Hearing Levels   77-81
  Auditory Training   83-86
  Checks of Function   86-88, 151
  Frequency Range   68-73
  Gain   65-67, 78-81
  Selection of   81-83, 149-151

-i-   139
i-e   145
Improvement of Speech   173-177
International Phonetic Alphabet   9-11
Intonation   34-35

j   127

k   99
Kinesthetic Information, Speech   25-26, 32

l   133
Language Development   43, 154-155
Learning Abilities   47-50
Loudness   186

m   128

Maintenance of Speech   190-192
Manner of Production   20-23
Methodology   54-57, 147-168, 174-177
  Association Phoneme Unit   163-166
  Auditory Global   148-159
  Choosing a Method   166-168
  Multisensory Syllable Unit   159-163
Multisensory Syllable Unit Method   159-163

n   130
Nasal Cavity   19-20
Nasality   30, 181, 184-185
  Feature Recognition   75-76
ng   131
Northampton Charts   12-13
Northampton Symbols   10-14

o-e   145
oi   145
Onset Characteristics, Phonemes   76
oo   141
oo   141
Oral Cavity   18
Oral Environment   51, 52-53
Orthographic Systems   8-15, 158
  Diacritical Markings   10-11
  International Phonetic Alphabet   9-11
  Northampton Symbols   10-14
  Visible Speech Symbols (Bell)   9
  Visual-Tactile System (Zaliouk)   9-10
ou   145

p   94
Palate   18
Perceptual Features, Speech
  Articulation   23-27
  Rhythm   39
  Voice   30-32
Phonation   29-30
Phoneme   7-8, 164-165
Phrasing   36
Physical Growth and Maturation   42-44
  Dental   16-17, 42
  Motor   42-43
Pitch   38
  Control of   186
  Fundamental   186
Place of Production   15-20, 21, 23
  Recognition of   76-77

qu   138

r   135
Rate, Speech   36-38
Reinforcement   56, 158
Repetition   56

Resonant Sounds 22
Resonation 30
Respiration 28-29
Rhythm 7, 32-39
  Features 33-39
    Accent 33-34
    Emphasis 34
    Intonation 34-35
    Perceptual Features of 38-39
    Phrasing 36
    Rate 36-38
  Irregularities of 186-190
  Production 32

s̜ 105
School Program 52-63
  Methodology 54-56
  School Oral Environment 52-53
  Sensory Channels and Aids 56-63
  Systematic Instruction 53-54
Sensation Level 78
Sensory Abilities 44-46
Sensory Aids 56-58, 60-63
Sensory Channels 56-63
Sensory Instructional Possibilities 26-27
  Tactile 27
  Visual 26-27
sh 108
Stops 20
Stridency 185-186
Student 42-50
  Learning Abilities 47-50
  Physical Growth and Maturation 42-44

Sensory Abilities 44-46
Syllable 32-33, 162-163

t 96
Tactile Information, Speech 24-27, 32, 160
t̩h 104
t̪h 122

-u- 142
u-e 145
ur 143

v 121
Visible Speech Symbols (Bell) 9
Vision, Disorders 44-45
Visual Information, Speech 26-27
Visual-Tactile System (Zaliouk) 9
Voice 7, 28-32
  Abnormalities of 183-186, 190
  Fundamental Frequency 29
  Harmonics of 30
  Loudness 186
  Perceptual Features of 30-32
  Pitch 186
  Production of 28-30
  Recognition of 74-75
  Resonation 30
Voicing 74-75

w 112
wh 93
x 138
y- 137
z 124
zh 125

DATE DUE

NOV 1 1 '76			
MAR 1 7 '77			
AUG 1 4 '77			
OCT 2 9 1981			
3/29/82			
SEP 1 5 1983			
JUL 2 5 1985			
SEP 8 1986			
DEC 1 1 1986			
NOV 1 2 1991			
FEB 1 1 1995			
NOV 2 8 1995			